T0381077

ADVANCED KENPO KARATE: THE WU SHEN PAI METHOD
VOLUME I: THE MASTER KEYS

By Professor Robert L. Jones

DEDICATION

To my wife, Kris. You are my life and my love! Thanks for the years we have had together. I hope to continue a long journey of many more years ahead with you both in our personal and professional lives. It has given me the greatest joy to give you that which I

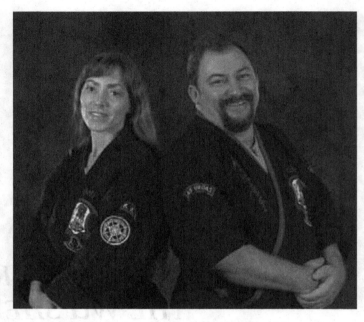

Sifu Jones and Sibok Jones

hold to be sacred, my skills and knowledge of Wu Shen Pai Kenpo and to see them blossom within you.

To my life coaches: To Barry Gruters who taught me that the most important thing in life was to love God with all my heart, mind, and spirit. And to Michael Howell-Moroney who showed me the way.

Sibok Robert L. Jones

Trafford
PUBLISHING® www.trafford.com

North America & international
toll-free: 844-688-6899 (USA & Canada)
fax: 812 355 4082

ACKNOWLEDGEMENTS

No work such as this occurs in a vacuum. There are many who have contributed both directly and indirectly to this work. First I want to acknowledge my dearest wife Kris, who has sacrificed much to the creation of the Wu Shen Pai Kenpo system, and who shares my love of the art. Without her unflagging support, this work would not have been possible. I would like to thank my instructors through the years in the arts of Jung Shin Do and American Kenpo. They have been talented and knowledgeable martial artists. I have learned over my journey through the martial way what it truly means to live with honor and dignity and to walk with confidence. I have also learned through these many years how to stand up for what I believe in, even when I am standing alone. The teachings gleaned from the arts of Jung Shin Do and American Kenpo have congealed into what I choose to term Wu Shen Pai Kenpo or "Martial Spirit Family" of Kenpo. I consider it a method or approach to the study of Kenpo which I have founded.

One person who has answered many questions for me and prompted many more is Sigung Antwione Alferos. He has made many contributions to my personal and professional development along the way in my Wu Shen Pai Kenpo journey. I would like to publicly thank Sigung Alferos for his support and friendship. He is a man of faith and iron integrity who has my respect and my affection. He is a mentor to me in many ways who has shown me how a master of the martial arts conducts himself.

I would like to thank my good friend and student Robert Austin for reviewing the final manuscript and for his many helpful post-production suggestions with printing and editing. I also owe him a debt of gratitude for his unflagging support of this project, and of Wu Shen Pai Kenpo in general. I am grateful to him most of all for his friendship and brotherhood. His positive leadership in the martial arts community and his willingness to make a contribution has been an inspiration to me and to all those who know him. I am proud to be associated with him. He is a largely unsung hero in the Kenpo and martial arts world for whom our entire martial arts community should be grateful. I want to thank him publicly for his countless contributions to my growth. He has taught me what truly matters in life, he has pushed me to greater accomplishment and has earned my gratitude, my respect, and my friendship. He has made me to think about the big picture of why we are here and what we hope to contribute more than any one in Kenpo. For that and much more besides, I feel I have been blessed with his friendship. Sibok Robert Austin is a true pioneer who teaches from the heart and who has been my friend for over 12 years. He has taught me as much, if not more than I have ever taught him.

I want to thank my students who have probably heard every aspect of this work in the developmental stages and who have helped me, and continue to help me, refine the ideas presented here. I am truly grateful for your input along the way. As with all teachers, my students are my greatest teachers.

Specifically, I wish to thank Sisook Ron Young and Sisook Mike Moser for their inspiration in the preparation of this project. I would like to acknowledge those who have helped in the preparation of this work by posing for the various illustrations used within the book. My thanks go out to my senior Black Belt students, Sifu Bob Burke and Sifu Kris Jones. I would also like to thank many other seniors who participated in this project: Sisook Sarah Bond Carter, Sisook Joshua Bond, Sisook Dustin Carter, Sisook Ashley Carter, Sisook Mark Weber, Sisook Rick Taylor, Sisook Joshua Bond and Sisook Jasmin Bond for their efforts in the support of this project. I am extremely proud to call these individuals Black Belts in every sense of the term. In addition to my Black Belts, I would also like to thank one of the other senior students who participated in the principal photography for this volume, Wosu Dennis Diaz, who tirelessly assisted me by posing for the photographic illustrations of techniques and Master Keys that appear in this volume and others. Thanks should also be extended to Mr. Jay Talcott of Solutions West Photography for his tireless efforts in shooting the photographs which appear in this book. He is a consummate professional whose friendship and assistance were invaluable in the preparation of this volume. I am grateful to Wosu Dennis Diaz for his tireless labor in the digital editing of the photographic work that appears in these volumes. It is truly great work!

Sibok Robert L. Jones
7th Degree Black Belt, American Wu Shen Pai Kenpo
International Kenpo Karate Society
February 20, 2005

FORWARD

The explanations of the art of Kenpo contained within this work are based upon the art of Wu Shen Pai Kenpo (or Chuan Fa) The Art of Wu Shen Pai Kenpo was founded on September 11, 2004. It was immediately recognized by the United States Martial Arts Association and the United Martial Arts Alliance. Both organizations conferred upon me a 7th Degree Black Belt and the title of "Hanshi" or "Master Teacher". Wu Shen Pai Kenpo is based on the theory of Yin and Yang or the unity of polar opposites. This theory states that in nature there is a co-existence of polar dichotomies. For every one, there is an equal opposite. For every concept, principle, theory, definition and movement in Wu Shen Pai Kenpo there is an opposite and a reverse. Wu Shen Pai Kenpo is a combination of Yin {soft/circular movement} and Yang {hard/linear movement}, making it one of the most diversified and comprehensive martial arts to be found in the world. Its study integrates the spiritual, mental, and physical disciplines enabling its practitioners to realize their full potential in all areas of life.

The Dynamics of *Wu Shen Pai*

Three Elements of Yin, the essence of **Wu Shen Pai Kenpo** soft techniques:
- *Liu* - soft, fluid force of flowing water. The power of Yu is deceptive and relenting under force; it draws its attack into its own stream of power and re-directs it.
- *Yuan* - is movement in circular directions. Its power may be seen in the rock at the end of a sling, or the power developed from a spinning motion.
- *He* - as the third element of Yin, it represents unity and combination.

Three Elements of *Yang*, the essence of **Wu Shen Pai Kenpo** hard techniques:
- *Gang* - is hard like steel or stone. Its power is illustrated in the form of a closed fist in a thrust punch or a straight front kick.
- *Jiao* - means angles. Its form is found in the correct angle of the joint when applying breaking and throwing techniques or straight angular blocks.
- *Jian* - means maintaining proper distance. It is the opposite aspect of He or combination and its form is found in understanding the distance between two opponents.

Wu Shen Pai Chuan Fa teaches both the martial art and healing art. If one is able to injure or kill, then he/she should know how to heal as well, once again maintaining harmony through balance of opposites. In the martial arts applications, Wu Shen Pai Kenpo is best understood by an examination of its four Divisions of Power. The martial applications of **Wu Shen Pai** can be further explained in four distinct, though interconnected, paths of study within the art.

NEI GUNG - deals with one's internal energy (Chi power) development, control and direction. Through both passive and active methods, Chi power development is taught via specialized breathing and meditation exercises in conjunction with specific physical exercises. The practitioner learns to develop, harness, and apply this human energy resource at will. Initially studied for health purposes and for use in the battlefield; at more advanced levels this power can be controlled in conjunction with mental processes and can be extended from one individual to another for healing as well as combative applications. This internal energy is found in all living creatures, yet in the disciplined study of Wu Shen Pai Kenpo one can learn to develop this power for truly outstanding displays of human energy and will, extending previously conceived limitations to unlimited possibilities. There are five different senses of Chi that may be developed:

- making the body light
- making the body heavy
- making the body hard as steel
- making the body numb
- increasing mental concentration and awareness

WEI GUNG – This takes its form in the offensive and defensive combative applications found within the art and is the externalization of Nei Gung. Most martial arts are either tense and linear in their orientation or are soft and circular. **Wu Shen Pai** combines both elements to form a natural and compatible combative system. This phase of instruction includes all forms of hand strikes and blocks (trapping and grabbing as well as deflection applications, using the hands, wrist, forearm, elbows, arms and shoulders): 365 individual kicks; throws and falls from any position and onto any surface; human anatomical structure/function as it pertains to combative applications (knowing and utilizing the body's weak points to effectively control the opponent, regardless of their size); joint manipulation and/or bone breaking; finger pressure point applications; containment, control, and transport techniques; grappling applications; forms; offensive choking/breaking techniques; defense against multiple assailants; counter-offense and defense for the above and additional advanced, secretive techniques. These applications are taught in their combative form, yet with full control in order to minimize danger to the student. By practicing these diverse aspects, one can regain and maintain health through physical exercise while learning to control any antagonist within one movement. **Wu Shen Pai** techniques are implemented to the degree a particular situation dictates, applying an incremental escalation of force.

WU CHI GUNG - involves the offensive and defensive use of the over 108 traditional weapons found within 20 categories of weaponry. By learning these various weapon systems, the practitioner can most effectively utilize any object as a weapon as the situation demands.

SHEN GUNG - is the study, develop, and control of the human mind in order to attain one's full potential and mental capabilities. Techniques are taught to achieve an increase in one's total awareness, focus, and concentration levels. This realm includes instruction in controlling one's mind, development of the "sixth sense", memory recall, understanding the natural laws of the universe, the study of human character and personalities, practical psychology, visualization, the art of concealment and stealth, as well as advanced, secretive applications. These powers and more lie within the potentials of every human being and can be developed and utilized through the proper training methods.

The healing arts aspects (the study of Traditional Chinese Medicine or the Oriental Healing Arts) of **Wu Shen Pai** are every bit as complex and demanding as the study of Occidental Medicine. The student of **Wu Shen Pai** learns to become one with the natural laws of the universe, learning all aspects of self-defense in an ever-changing environment. These defensive applications can apply on a basic level, such as close quarter combatives, as well as on a more intricate level of healing injuries and disease. Therefore, in order to most effectively defend oneself from these outside elements, the practitioners of **Wu Shen Pai** learns to develop the capacity to heal themselves as well as others. First aid applications and revival techniques are taught in conjunction with the traditional full studies of acupuncture, acupressure, herbal and natural medicines, and bone setting or body manipulation.

On a more mundane level, this Division of Power refers to the study of the Concepts and Principles of the art. The understanding of the natural laws of physics and the Master Keys of the art that enable a practitioner to train more efficiently.

For further information on Wu Shen Pai Kenpo or its governing body, the International Kenpo Karate Society, please visit the Association website at http://www.ikkskenpo.com or you may email me at info@ikkskenpo.com

Senior Professor Robert L. Jones,
7th Degree Black Belt, International Kenpo Karate Society
Founder, Wu Shen Pai Kenpo system

INTRODUCTION

Senior Grandmaster Ed Parker, the founder of American Kenpo, at one point queried a group of black belt instructors "If a man crosses the street and is hit by a garbage truck, which part of the truck hits the man first?" Those in the seminar, many of them high-ranking blacks belts, suggested various possible responses such as "the bumper", "the grill", or "the tires". Some considered the possibility that Mr. Parker was asking a trick question of some sort. He was not. The answer, to be succinct, is just what Ed Parker suggested it would be. After hearing all of the various responses, he retorted that the man would be hit by "the whole truck".

The point of this exercise was the easy analogy which one could draw between the hitting power of the Kenpo system and the hitting power of the truck. If the truck truly could separate its various components and hit with only its bumper, its grill, or its tires, it would be severely constraining its potential power. The reason the truck hits so hard is precisely because it hits with all of these possible elements. The human body, like the truck, is constrained by the laws of physics which dictate that certain conditions must be met to maximize our efficiency in motion. With all elements in place, these same laws of physics also dictate that power is maximized. With minimum effort, then, greater efficiency in motion is obtained. For those who are seriously engaged in the study of the martial arts, this is the eternal quest, maximum efficiency with minimum effort. It is particularly true of American Wu Shen Pai Kenpo Karate

practitioners that we are ever engaged in the search for greater efficiency in our

motion. This may be why the history of Kenpo has been one of adaptation and

change. As many have wryly observed, Kenpo never changes, it is in a perpetual

state of refinement. American Kenpo is the predecessor to our system of Wu

Shen Pai Kenpo. Our system is a further refinement of that art. This refinement

has been in constant search of methods of execution that would serve to give the

Kenpo practitioner greater speed and hitting power. These are the elusive

components that all martial artists seek in order to improve the physical

constituents of their arts. The strength of American Wu Shen Pai Kenpo is that

its basis lies in physical laws to which all humans beings are subject. These laws

have seldom been elaborated upon before, and aside from Wu Shen Pai Kenpo's

ingenious adaptation of physics, have never been used to explain motion

inherent to the martial arts. In fact, the continual refinement of the American Wu

Shen Pai Kenpo system lie in its search for an overarching method to further

advance our study, the study of motion.

The purpose of this book is to aid the student of Kenpo Karate in

understanding the various types of Master Keys, the concepts, theories, basics,

and techniques which will enhance the understanding of the laws of physics

upon which Kenpo, and all martial arts, depend for obtaining power and

maximizing efficiency. It is hoped that, with diligent application of the

principles discussed in this book, higher levels of skill in Kenpo might be obtained. The aim of this work is to raise the standards of skill and excellence in American Wu Shen Pai Kenpo, and in the martial arts as a whole if they might derive some lessons from our system. By applying the principles discussed within this work, it is possible to enhance efficiency, speed, and the overall development of skill training within our art such that Kenpo might indeed be about "**overskill**" and not about **overkill**. It is to aid in the development of the entire Kenpo community that this work is humbly offered to all Kenpo practitioners. But within a larger context, the Master Keys discussed in this work are universal, applicable to all martial arts systems, and hence may aid all martial artists in seeking to better understand their art.

He who knows **how** will always be the student, while he who knows **why** will always be the instructor. It is my hope that this work will be but one contribution to deepening our understanding of "why". It is also my hope that the work contained within this volume will in some sense serve the next generation of Wu Shen Pai Kenpo practitioners as a foundation upon which other and deeper understandings of the principles and concepts which form the core of our art are better established. Moreover, it is hoped that all martial arts and martial artists may benefit from this work.

In the world of science, newer paradigms, or systems of knowledge, replace older paradigms as the newer paradigms examine more phenomena not successfully explained by the older paradigm. For example, in the world of physics, Newton discovered laws, now systematized as Newtonian mechanics, which apply to the planetary spheres of discovery. Einstein subsequently theorized about the very large and the very fast and provided us with the basis of our modern understanding of the universe and space travel. Quantum physics is the new frontier of that branch of science which explores the very small. Each might be seen as limiting instances of one great branch of science known as physics. Currently physics gropes for a unifying field theory that will serve to unite all of these realms within the discipline. It is my hope that the theories of Wu Shen Pai Kenpo might make similar breakthroughs possible for the martial arts. Until recently, Kenpo has been understood in terms of its Newtonian Mechanics. It is my hope that further exploration of the topics within this book will make possible a new frontier in the exploration of concepts and principles of motion within a micro context, hence leading to a "Quantum Kenpo" of sorts. Further, I would hope that the principles elaborated upon in this work, macro and micro, might be universal in character. This is what I hoped for in the development of the Wu Shen Pai Kenpo system, that it would lead the way toward principles that would aid the practitioners of all martial arts, no matter the style.

The basis of this multi-volume work is to introduce the student to the Master Keys, explore advanced concepts, and boldly examine the new frontiers in the evolution of my own system of Kenpo which I term Wu Shen Pai Kenpo, control manipulation and pressure point theory. I will explore within the first volume the **Physical, Emotional, Spiritual,** and **Mental Master Keys**.

Specifically, I will explain, define, and elaborate upon the **Physical Master Keys**, or the **Master Key Basics, Techniques, Forms, Sets, Movements, Timing Patterns, Control Manipulations, Positions, Motion Patterns**, and **Methods of Execution**. Additionally I will explore the **Master Key Concepts**, or **Mental Master Keys** which would include **Economy of Motion, Meeting Force, the Presence and Use of Physical Master Keys, Anatomical Positioning, Point of Origin**, and **Timing for Effect**. **Master Key Theories** will also be assessed including the **Power Equations, Family Groupings**, and **Master Key Strategies** for dealing with an attack. **Spiritual Master Keys** include **being at peace with those around you, being at peace with yourself, and having confidence in yourself.**

The bio-mechanical basis of this work is a very simple physics formula taught at every high school in the nation. This understanding, unfortunately, is seldom applied to the martial arts outside of Wu Shen Pai Kenpo. This formula is

$$\sum \tfrac{1}{2} (M) (V)^2 = \text{Force. Where } M = \sum [(rm) (vm) (hm)] \text{ PBA.}$$

Or stated more succinctly, where **mass is the sum of rotational momentum, horizontal momentum, and vertical momentum, multiplied by Proper Body Alignment**. Proper Body Alignment is in turn defined as the subset of physiological engagement multiplied by the forward projection of our weight. Stated mathematically PBA = [(fp) (pe)]. These factors are aided by our able employment of our zones of offense. Our velocity is defined as V= [(r) (d) (t)]^2 where rate is the rate of speed (or physical speed of our motion), distance is the distance to the target and time is the time it takes us to travel to the target at our constant speed. This is squared. Put another way, our velocity is defined in terms of our physical speed, which is enhanced by increasing our speed of execution to the main target.

There are a number of ways to achieve this increase in speed. One of these methods of obtaining increased velocity is through a principle termed "elastic recoil." Another method is to round off the corners and elongate our circles which lead us to cut the distance to the target. Still another method of increasing speed most commonly used in kicking and striking is through the employment of a principle termed "Circumferential Acceleration." There is also "Circular Compression" through which an increase in speed is achieved. Most significantly, there is a fourth method of increasing speed that is often overlooked. This method is inherent in such principles as meeting force and entails taking full advantage of the opponent's anticipated response to our various strikes such that he (or she) will actually move physically toward the strike itself. By employing this principle, the opponent actually aids us by moving toward us thus decreasing the distance to target. It is my hope to more fully elaborate on the element of speed in American Wu Shen Pai Kenpo than has previously been the case in any previous work on the subject. As the chapter which further explores these equations will show, there is a complex web of relationships which is best articulated through the vehicle of mathematics. The hope is that by more fully exploring these relationships, we may more fully appreciate how best to train ourselves and our students to maximize our potential.

The relationship of each element in these equations is interwoven so tightly and each of these principles and concepts is so interdependent that a failure to apply one principle to the fullest may adversely impact the power achieved by a factor much larger than the importance of that factor taken by itself may indicate. In other words, these complex elements, taken together, have a synergy which far exceeds their individual importance. By way of illustration, we might look to the impact which our Body Attitude, with respect to the opponent, has when we over rotate or place our body outside of its appropriate relationship. We lose Proper Body Alignment in this instance through over rotation. The Angle of Scaption is also lost which means that our physical speed to target decreases. As this occurs, we lose power by a factor of four. We also lose Three Dimensional Hitting as we lose Body Attitude which derives from the limits that over-rotation place on our ability to utilize Rotational Momentum, Vertical Momentum, and Horizontal Momentum in direct application of our mass to the target. We lose maximum impact potential as we move past the forty-five degree angle. There are myriad other concepts and principles we lose the ability to bring to the table when we lose body attitude, all of which might help us obtain greater power through mass or speed.

There are those who might question the forthright discussion of principles utilizing terms which Edmund K Parker, the Senior Grandmaster and founder of American Kenpo, never utilized in his teaching career. I believe it is reasonable to suggest that these terms, concepts, and theories as they are expressed herein are logical evolutions of existing concepts, theories, definitions, and principles which were used by Senior Grandmaster Ed Parker at various times. There are, however, many aspects of the study of the concepts and principles of American Kenpo which were still in the exploration stage at the time of Mr. Parker's untimely death. I address these areas in my own study and teaching of American Wu Shen Pai Kenpo in my own way and do not allege that Ed Parker used these terms in any way. In addition to concepts, theories and definitions which are based upon concepts which Mr. Parker propounded during his lifetime, there are also terms that I employ which are wholly my own. These terms, however, are logical extensions of concepts, principles, theories, and definitions which the Senior Grandmaster expressed at times. My own self-expression of these concepts stems from an effort to derive agreement within an extremely diverse range of Martial Arts, and Kenpo, training theories. I have been blessed with a broad exposure to a wide range of thought within Kenpo and seek agreement, truth, and unity in diversity. This diversity of thought and training theories finds its unity in my system of Wu Shen Pai Kenpo (or Chuan Fa) The concepts addressed in this book, in my view, are in harmony with the Kenpo that the Senior Grandmaster taught in my experience. I cannot speak to any other training experience with Senior Grandmaster Ed Parker, only my own. Therefore no attempt is made to do so. I believe that the goal of furthering our progress and our training in the art of Kenpo, Edmund K. Parker's life work, would be one that Mr. Parker would unhesitatingly embrace. I also feel that any work that serves to aid a student or instructor in bettering their own interpretation of Kenpo is beneficial as it is clear that all beneficial efforts, no matter how minor, lead to ultimate perfection. It is my hope that this book, while certainly addressing the concerns of those within every form of Kenpo may also reach out to a broader audience within the martial arts community. It is my hope that the Master Keys and other universal principles that are introduced to the student of American Wu Shen Pai Kenpo, when given wider exposure, might serve as a "Rosetta stone" of sorts which enable us to decode motion on a broader scale. With this in mind, our system may be of great benefit in improving the execution of technique in all martial artists regardless of their chosen discipline. My motive is simply to contribute to the growth and progress of those in the martial arts.

Senior Grandmaster Ed Parker suggested that the system of American Kenpo would continue to grow, evolve, and develop. This is indeed what American Wu Shen Pai system represents. It is an evolution of the American Kenpo System and of my earlier martial arts experiences that broadened and deepened my own understanding of Kenpo from the very first. Clearly, this new Kenpo system stands on the shoulders of those systems that have gone before,

American Kenpo and Jung Shin Do. I liken this process to that of the academic world, in which an accumulation of knowledge occurs over the years which leads to evolution in, for example, physics. The discipline remains the constant, it is our expression of it that may change or alter to fit new theories and understandings of our natural world. In American Wu Shen Pai Kenpo terms, the alphabet of motion does not change, although the manner in which we may use it does. We could easily agree that, as adults, none of us writes or understands our grammar in the same way that we did in grade school. Thus, our expression of the written alphabet has changed and grown more sophisticated. The alphabet has not been altered because, in some nebulous fashion, the letter "Z" "did not work" for us. Rather, we had best retain the letter "Z" in the unlikely event we would wish to spell the word "zebra". Such a task would prove impossible for those without the letter "Z" in their alphabet. When the view is expressed that a given technique does not work, usually it is because some principles for the application of that technique is lacking the training of that individual. For whom does a technique not work effectively? It is my view that Kenpo techniques should be universal in character. That is that they might be effectively worked by anyone on anyone. This obviously does not mean that the art does not grow and evolve within the individual thus making the art more efficient to that individual. The art as a whole should also continue to grow and evolve. This is the essence of what American Wu Shen Pai Kenpo is all about. It brings elements into play that, literally, complete the art of Kenpo. These are elements that have been noted as being absent by some of the more accomplished practitioners of Kenpo. Our system, however, continues to be one that would literally wrap itself around the practitioner and ultimately lead to an expression that is unique to that individual. There are signatures of motion, to be sure, but the expression of that signature itself is unique. This is our perception of what "style" was. We perceive style as a method of expressing our system. A system is something very much like unto an alphabet. It remains fixed while we might employ block printing, cursive writing, or even shorthand in our expressive style, the constants remain the alphabet with which we work to express ourselves. We might choose another alphabet and then alter our expression of even that alphabet, but the alphabets for the language of motion remain as the constant. It is only when we attempt to alter the alphabet by cutting the number of letters and then express ourselves, that we find that we have something less than before. A system, in other words changes ever so rarely and then only when those who thoroughly understand it take the evolution of that system to the next level. I believe that the key to the growth and progress of the martial arts consists of teaching your students correct principles and then allowing those principles to govern their motion. This would result in the growth and evolution of that student in terms of their expression of the system. The system vocabulary would expand with the evolution of Wu Shen Pai allowing for variable expansion and force continuums previously unexplored. Wu Shen Pai Kenpo evolves Kenpo into the future by teaching self-defense from disadvantaged positions, exploring a systematic curriculum in the healing arts, pressure points, and joint manipulation. This work began as a single volume and ultimately grew to a three-volume set. The first volume considers the Master Keys in their various forms. The second volume will discuss the various aspects of contact manipulation and control maintenance that are integral to our system of American Wu Shen Pai Kenpo. The third volume will bring to light the pressure point and cavity press theories that are also integral to the American Wu Shen Pai Kenpo system.

It is my view that the Kenpo system is an extraordinary one. I believe that it is based on patterns of motion and immutable laws that are merely communicated through the vehicle of our Wu Shen Pai Kenpo System. Wu Shen Pai Kenpo communicates the discovery of these laws of physics and motion through categorization and systemization of the laws of motion. There are natural and immutable laws of motion and physics that exist independently of our belief in or knowledge of them. The patterns that we acknowledge as valid in American Wu Shen Pai Kenpo communicate to us how those laws may be intelligently utilized in defending ourselves and fulfilling our lives. Wu Shen Pai Kenpo taps into these natural laws and expresses them in physical terms. There might be those who would suggest that I am reading far too much into the simplicity that is Kenpo Karate. To those who would make this criticism I can only say that I do not believe in coincidence. I certainly do not believe that the number of coincidences necessary for all of this to be true might come about naturally. Much of that which is Wu Shen Pai Kenpo utilizes the syllabus of American Kenpo because there are patterns of regularity in the Kenpo system, and consequently within the art of Wu Shen Pai Kenpo Karate, awaiting discovery. Whether they are present in the system due to coincidence or through design is irrelevant in the final analysis. Who has generated the analysis that yields them is irrelevant as well. Truth discovered remains true regardless of who the discoverer might be. The knower exists independently of that which is known. What counts only is the presence or absence of these patterns or truths about motion. It is my hope that, at the very least, this work will point the way to other creative conceptions about our system. My opinions about the Kenpo system and the martial arts in general are, in the end, what this work is all about. But, this is true of all academic examinations of any subject. Ultimately this work is my own synthesis, my own analysis, and I alone bear the full responsibility for any errors that it may contain. You may choose to agree or disagree with the contents of this book, and that is the essence of free inquiry. However, I offer this work on my system of Kenpo Karate as my own humble contribution to the literature on the martial arts. It is my hope that others will take the concepts expressed herein and build upon them, should they choose to do so. It is clearly the case that this work stands on the shoulders of many others who have contributed to the evolution of our system through its almost 50 years of existence here in the United States. It is also true that American Kenpo rests on older systems of Kung Fu that date back to about 344 A.D. Knowledge never spontaneously generates. It is always an outgrowth of what has gone before. It is important, and honorable, to acknowledge that. At the very least this work will generate discussion, the greatest vehicle for learning and growth.

With thanks to all those who have gone before and particularly to Senior Grandmaster Edmund K. Parker, on whose shoulder we stand. Our system of Wu Shen Pai Kenpo Karate is a further elaboration of, or formulation of, the American Kenpo system. It fully encompasses that art while filling in the gaps in that knowledge base. It is my view that this is the direction in which American Kenpo was intended to go. Ed Parker, in my view, fully intended that his Black Belts be knowledgeable in the traditional Chinese healing arts, in pressure point and cavity press theory, and in the joint manipulations which we utilize at the contact manipulation and control maintenance ranges. May the current and future generations of American Wu Shen Pai Kenpo practitioners be the ultimate beneficiaries of these efforts.

Chapter One

Physical Constituents of Power: Master Key Basics

There has been much discussion and little agreement in Kenpo Karate when the question of Master Keys is assessed. Perhaps the best way to reconcile the divergent viewpoints on Master Keys would be to suggest that there are several different types of Master Keys. On the whole, they share the characteristics of providing many answers within a single move or sequence of moves. One could reasonably assert that there are **Physical, Emotional, Spiritual** and **Mental Master Keys**.

In terms of **Physical Master Keys**, there are **Master Key Basics, Techniques, Forms, Sets, Movements, Timing Patterns, Techniques, Control Manipulations, Positions, Patterns,** and **Methods of Execution.**

Additionally there are **Master Key Concepts** without which it may even be asserted that Wu Shen Pai Kenpo, or any other form of Kenpo Karate, is not being practiced. These **Mental Master Keys** would include **Economy of Motion, Meeting Force, the Presence and Use of Physical Master Keys, Anatomical Positioning, Point of Origin,** and **Timing for Effect. Master Key Theories** include the **Power Equations, Family Groupings,** and also **Master Key Strategies** for dealing with an attack. **Master Key Tactics** may also be assessed within the category of **Mental Master Keys**.

Spiritual Master Keys at the first level include **being at peace with those around you (Peace Without), being at peace with yourself (Peace Within), and having confidence in yourself.** All of these are rooted in the self esteem of the practitioner.

When we consider Physical Master Keys and their many forms, they connect at one place. The root of all Physical Master Keys lies in the Master Key Basics.

Master Key Basics - Stances

Master Key Basics are primarily taught to beginning students and include the Inward Block or the Neutral Bow and Arrow stance. These are the individual movements, or stances, blocks, parries, punches, strikes, finger techniques, kicks, and foot maneuvers which taken individually may still serve a variety of functions. Within the category of **Stances**, there are two Master Key Basics. The first is the **Neutral Bow and Arrow Neutral** or **Bow** stance. Figure 1 illustrates a proper Neutral Bow. When properly executed it leads to the state of being neutral with respect to the opponent. This position is always relative in terms of the defender and the opponent. It requires that we maintain the shoulders and hips in a forty-five degree angle relative to the opponent. This enables both the hips and the shoulders to operate within their proper range of action which we term "the

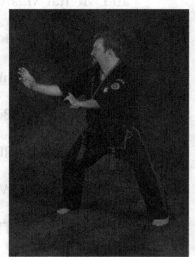

Figure 1

24

angle of scaption." This angle, when maintained, enables physiological engagement. This stance is tailored, through a heel-knee alignment to define proper depth which is illustrated in figure 2, at right. A toe-heel alignment defines proper width as illustrated in figure 3. Bending the knees to a comfortable level defines proper height. What makes this a master key basic is not only the multitude of uses that the stance enjoys, but also the fact that almost all other stances are built upon it.

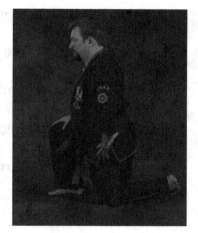

Figure 2

By way of illustration, the Forward Bow is executed from a Neutral and is properly tailored when the Neutral Bow is tailored properly. This is also true of the Reverse Bow, the Twist Stance, the Rotating Twist, the Horse, the Inverted Neutral Bow, and other less obvious views of the stance such as the Training Horse, Fighting Horse, Concave, and Diamond stances. It is easy to observe the same toe-heel relationship evidenced in the Neutral Bow also displayed in the Forward Bow. Figure 4 illustrates the same width relationship that we observe in the Neutral Bow. Since the Neutral Bow is tailored in this fashion, minor adjustment of the feet and establishing a Bracing Angle with the rear leg and Forward Projection with the forward leg does not alter the width

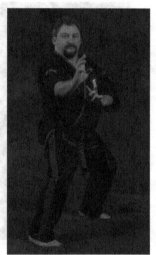

Figure 3

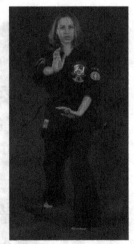

Figure 4

or the depth of the Forward Bow.

The Cat Stance is considered a transitional stance as is the One Leg stance. The Forward Bow and Arrow Stance of American Wu Shen Pai Kenpo visualized from a number of angles is illustrated below in figure 5. Figure 6 examines the Reverse Bow and Arrow stance, identical except in orientation, to the Forward Bow.

Figure 5

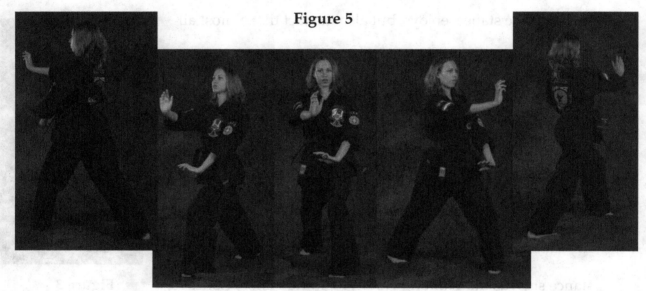

Figure 6

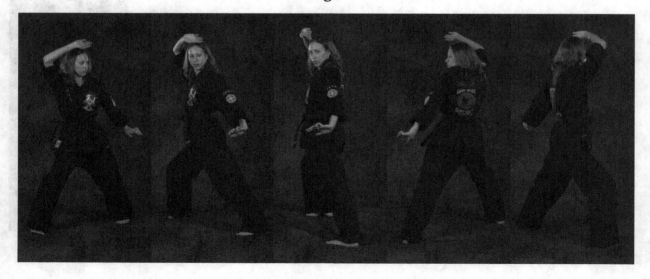

Aside from the Neutral Bow and Arrow Stance, the other Master Key Stance is the **Forward Bow and Arrow**. Although tailoring is accomplished for the Forward Bow from the Neutral Bow, it is different enough to be considered a **Master Key** basic in its own rite. This stance is the position on which the Close Kneel Stance is based, as is the Wide Kneel Stance. It is identical physically to the Reverse Bow, as noted above except with respect to orientation. Figure 7 illustrates the Wide Kneel from a variety of perspectives.

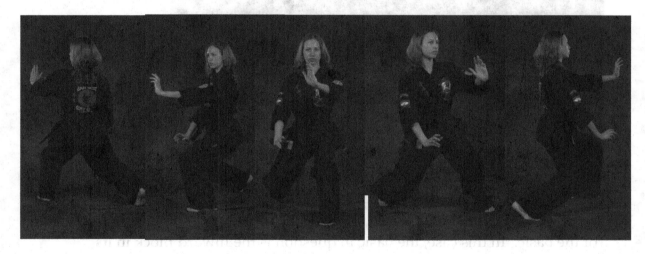

Figure 7

Master Key Basics - Blocks

Within the **category of Blocks**, there are **six Master Key Basics**. These are the **Inward, Vertical Outward, Extended Outward, Upward, Downward, and Push Down Blocks**. These blocks may be understood as Master Keys in the sense that they answer a variety of situations and dilemmas as blocks but also provide solutions as strikes. This sheds further light on the oft held axiom that a strike is a block and a block is a strike. We may seek, in other words, to redefine a basic more commonly known to us as a block. One example of this would be the Back Knuckle Rake which differs from the Inward Block only in terms of depth of penetration and intent. Figure 8 below illustrates the concept of redefining

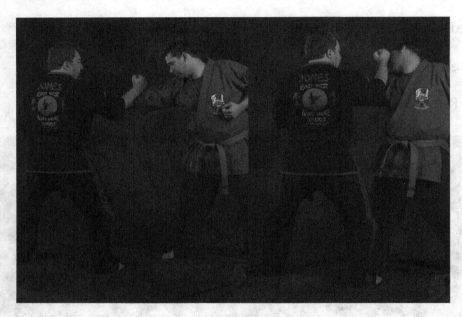

Figure 8

of the basic. In this case, the basic in question is the Inward Block in its relationship to the Back Knuckle Rake. They show that there is absolutely no physical difference in the actual execution of the two movements. Typically there is a step back with the execution of an Inward Block while in executing an Inward Back Knuckle Rake there is a step forward. Hence the only real difference between the two would be depth of penetration and intent. Another such example would involve the redefinition of the upward block as an upward forearm strike. Once again, as in the case of the Inward Block/Inward Back

Knuckle Rake, the physical execution of the basic in either blocking or striking modes is identical.

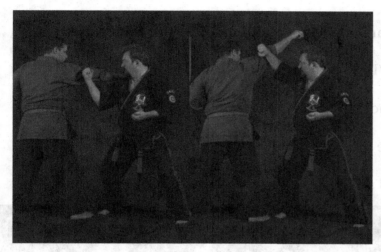

Figure 9

Figure 9 illustrates the use of the Upward Block as a blocking action. Figure 9 shows the initiation of the block through the fully extended blocking position. Figures 10 illustrates the use of this basic as an Upward Forearm Strike. This application of the basic offensively follows from its use in Long Form Two.

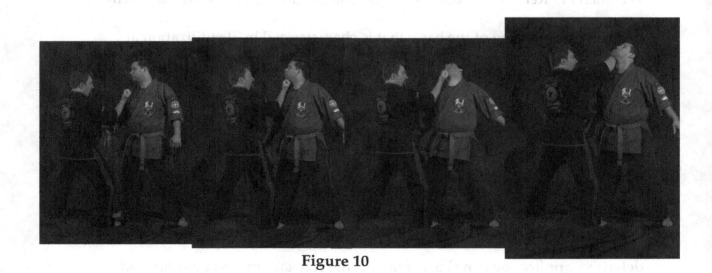

Figure 10

It follows that we might re-define the same motion in different ways much as we might re-define words which are spelled in similar ways but which, when placed in a different context, are applied in a different way. In this connection we might consider the word "light" which might be used to refer, alternately, to either weight or level of contact. The usage or context determines the meaning of the word. In figure 11, we see the application of the Vertical Outward Block. In these illustrations, the basic is utilized as a parrying block as it might be in the

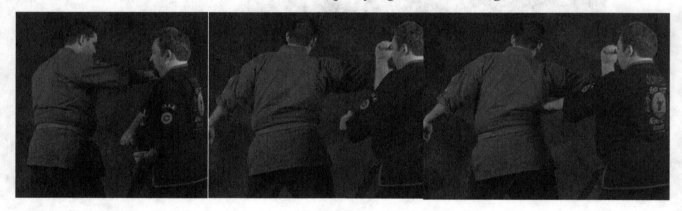

Figure 11

Wu Shen Pai Kenpo Blue Belt technique Shield and Mace. This is the strictly defensive application of the basic that is characterized by its utilization at medium or In Contact Range.

The Vertical Outward Block is then illustrated in figure 12 utilized as an Outward Back Knuckle Rake. This is the offensive application of the basic that is characterized by its use at close or Contact Penetration Range. Conversely it also represents the reverse motion of the Inward Block. Whether in its offensive or defensive applications, the basic remains the constant in the equation, and consequently the Master Key, since its utilization as a solution to a multitude of

dilemmas places it within that context.

Figure 12

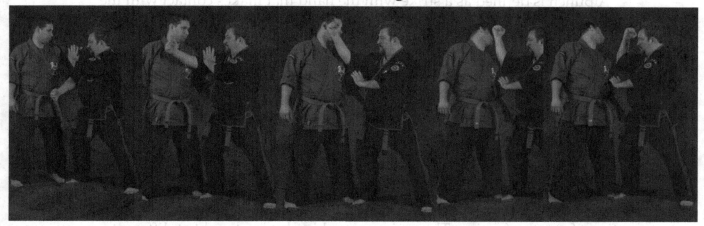

Master Key Basics - Parries

In the category of **Parries**, there are **Inward, Outward, Upward, and

Downward** parries that are Master Keys. Figure 13 shows, from left to right, an

Inward Parry, an Outward Parry from two perspectives, an Upward Parry, and a

Downward Parry.

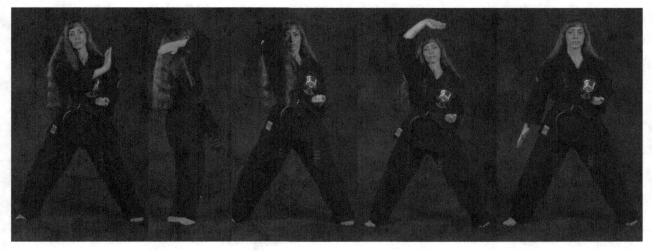

Figure 13

Master Key Basics - Punches

A punch is defined as a strike with the hand that makes contact with the target utilizing the frontal knuckles as the striking surface. Although physically defined in terms of contact with the knuckles of the hand to the target, truly all of the Punching techniques taught in the American Wu Shen Pai Yellow Belt curriculum are defined as being Master Key Basics. The execution of motion within the Punching category of the basics is better understood in terms of the execution of a path of action. The various punching basics, taught at different levels, become different points on that path. The Vertical Punch, under this view is merely an intermediate step between two other Master Key Basics, the Inverted Punch and the Straight Thrust Punch. The horizontal back knuckle is merely an inverted ordering of the vertical punch where the elbow is pointed and the fist follows rather than leads the action. All punching in American Kenpo might be viewed as simply points of contact along a path of action illustrated below. There is, in other terms, a relationship between and among these Master Key Basics. They are related by the fact that they share a path of action.

Although we might also understand the Inverted Punch as the Master Key **TO** punching, it is important to draw the distinction between this and **A** Master Key Punch such as the Straight Thrust Punch. The distinction between the two is this. The **Master Key TO Punching** is a **root word** of sorts. All punching, no matter what type, method, or manner of expression, must initiate through this phase of motion. A **Master Key Punch** is a basic that serves to illustrate for us one of several **Master Key Methods of Execution**.

The sequence of photos below in **Figures 14 and 15** illustrates the path of action, when viewed from the side, of the various punching basics taught in the Yellow Belt through Blue Belt Curriculum in Wu Shen Pai Kenpo. The **Master Key for Punching** starts the sequence and is taught as the **Inverted Punch**. Following this, the **Vertical Punch** is taught and followed by the **Straight Thrust Punch**. At full extension, the arm and hand turn inward and become first a **Roundhouse Punch**, then an **Inverted Vertical Roundhouse Punch**, and finally a **Hook Punch** and a **Looping Overhead Punch**. A **Back Knuckle Punch** and **an Inverted Back Knuckle Punch** are both part of this path of action. All of these are Master Key Basics taught at various levels. We can see this relationship spatially when we view this sequence from the side as in the figure below.

Figure 14

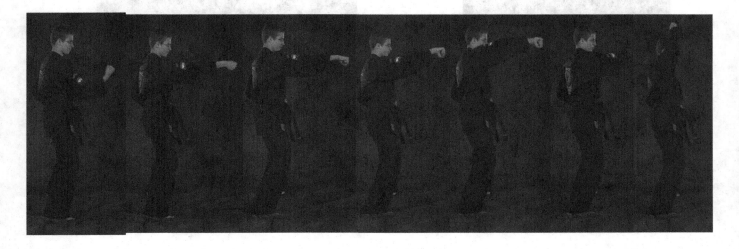

The **Hook Punch** becomes a point on the line of execution to an **Inverted Back Knuckle Strike**. This relationship is illustrated in Figure 15 below. In the punching path of action, the arm finally alters its path of action to become a **Looping Overhead Punch.** The cocking action at the embryonic level for a **Horizontal Back Knuckle** is the ending action for an **Inward Elbow Strike.** This relationship is shown by Figure 16 below. While an **Inward Elbow Strike** is nothing more than a **Hook Punch** that missed the mark. Punches and strikes are characterized, as we can see, by their interrelationships along paths and lines of action.

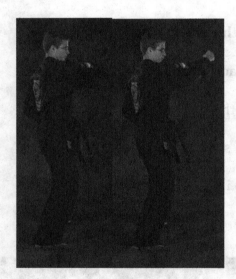
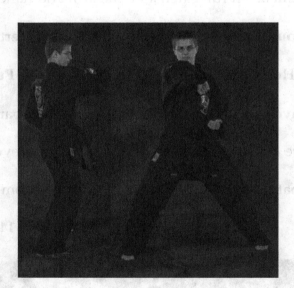

Figure 15   **Figure 16**

Master Key Basics - Strikes

It is important to note that there are **Master Key Strikes** within the **Master Key Basics**. Some of what is taught within this category is merely a redundancy in that there are some movements that replicate motion already modeled within other categories of **Master Key Basics**. A **Straight Heel Palm**, by way of illustration is merely a Straight Thrust Punch with a different natural weapon employed for the strike. An **Inward Handsword** is an **Inward Block** with the open hand, while an **Outward Handsword** is an **Extended Outward Block** with the open hand. In the category of **Strikes**, the Master Key Basics are **Inward, Outward, Upward,** and **Downward Elbow** Strikes. The **Inward** and **Upward Elbow Strike** as **Master Key Basics** and the **Outward Horizontal Elbow Strike** are illustrated in Figure 17.

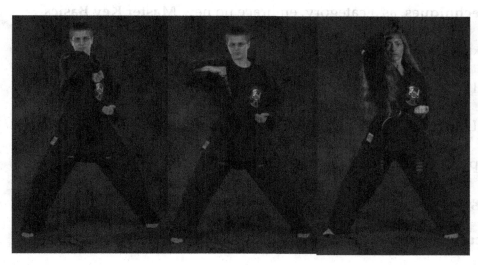

Figure 17

While An **Inward Horizontal Elbow Strike** is a "punch that missed", An **Outward Horizontal Elbow Strike** is the **Master Key Basic** for such fundamental movements as a **Back Elbow Strike** that is used extensively throughout the Kenpo System. Figure 18, on the following page, shows two possible applications of the **Inward** and **Outward Horizontal Elbow Strike**.

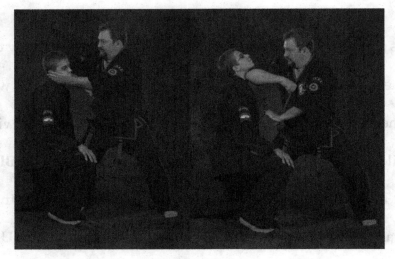

Figure 18

Master Key Basics – Finger Techniques

Finger Techniques, as a category, embrace no new **Master Key Basics**

since they are expressions of the same **Master Key Basics** while employing

different natural weapons. For example, the **Straight Finger Thrust** employed at

the Yellow Belt Level is merely a **Straight Thrust Punch** employing the fingers as

the natural weapons. The **Inward Overhead Claw** is merely an **Inward Block**

utilizing the fingers as the natural weapons expressed through the **Hammering**

Method of Execution. Even the **Inverted Vertical Claw**, taught at Orange Belt is

merely the Inverted Punch utilizing the fingers as the natural weapons and

employing the **Master Key Method of Execution** known as **Lift**.

Master Key Basics - Kicks

Kicking skills broadly entail, in Wu Shen Pai Kenpo as in other styles and

systems of martial arts, the use of the leg or foot to strike or impact the opponent.

What is unique to Wu Shen Pai Kenpo is that we subject kicking skills and body maneuvers to the same rigorous analysis to which we subject the motion of the

upper body. We should be able to identify the concepts and principles of

motion, as they apply to the lower body, through this analysis. The taxonomy or

categories of kicking techniques are broken down into three distinct types. There

are Snap Kicks, Thrust Kicks, and Circular Kicks among the 365 different kicks

utilized in Wu Shen Pai Kenpo.

When we speak of **Kicks** as **Master Key Basics**, we might more properly

be thinking in terms of first, the **Master Key For Kicking**, and second, of the

Master Key Kicking Basics. We might more properly understand the **Master**

Key Kicks, in other words, in terms of further categorical

breakdown. There is, first, the **Master Key FOR Kicking**

that is illustrated at right in Figure 19. This is so termed

because the position is the primary cocking position for all

kicking. Put another way, all kicking begins here. Figure 19

shows the **Master Key FOR Kicking** and the **Upward Knee**

Kick which is merely the Master Key for Kicking utilized as

a foot and leg strike. The rear leg roundhouse for example,

after establishing Center Point Balance is initiated from this

position, as is the front snap ball kick. Although the

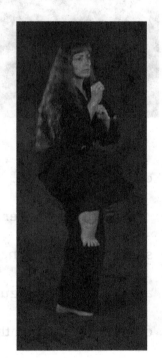

Figure 19

front leg snap roundhouse is initiated from what might be construed as a

different position illustrated in Figure 20, you will note that this position is

merely a variant of the position shown in Figure 19. As we closely look at Figure

20, below, we can see that this position is merely the same position angled off to forty-five degrees. Figure 20 illustrates the **Inward Knee Strike** and the **Secondary Master Key FOR Kicking.** A second variant of this coiled and ready position is shown in Figure 21. This is another **Secondary Master Key FOR**

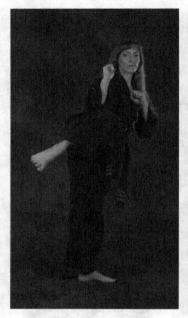 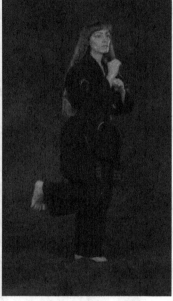

Kicking and a **Downward Knee Strike** in Figure 21. The initiation position for the **Back Snap** or **Back Thrust Kick** is shown in figure 21 at left. This, as can readily be observed, is the same preparatory position of

Figure 20   **Figure 21**   the leg with the knee pointed

directly downward.

   Kicking Master Key Basics might be referred to in order to master kicking skills since all kicking movements stem from these four **Master Key Kicks** which are illustrated in Figures 22 through 24. The **Master Key FOR Kicking** is most often utilized when the kick to be delivered is executed on a vertical plane and directed forward. The **Secondary Master Key FOR Kicking** shown in Figure 20 is most often utilized when the kick to be delivered is executed on a horizontal or forty-five degree diagonal plane of action or angle of execution and is directed forward or to the flank. The **Secondary Master Key FOR Kicking** illustrated in

Figure 21 is most often utilized when the kick to be delivered is executed on a vertical plane directed to the rear.

The **Primary Master Keys for Kicking** employ the **Inward, Outward, Upward, and Downward Knee Strike**, yet do not specifically focus on these strikes as kicks in the execution of basics. The execution of these **Master Keys for Kicking** might be thought of in terms of the execution of a Knee Strike in Inward, Outward, Upward, or Downward directions. Even when they are thought of in this way, they should properly be considered **the Primary and Secondary Master Keys for Kicking**. These basics might also be thought of as steps to achieving the full expression of the basics for which these Knee Strikes constituted the root words.

Master Key Kicks are the **four physical types of kicks** that are the foundational kicks for all kicking skill development. These are the **Front Snap Ball Kick**, the **Chop Kick**, the **Back Kick**, and **Side Knife Edge Kick**. All other kicks are merely variants of these four kicks. There are thrusting variants of the Master Key Kicks that are the **Front Thrust Kick, Roundhouse Kick, Side Thrust Kick**, and the **Back Thrust Kick**. Even within the third categorization of kicking techniques, Circular Kicks there are relationships existing between and among the Master Key Kicks. For example, a **Hook Kick** is the expression of the reverse motion of the **Roundhouse Kick**. Sweeps are the reverse motion of the **Side Knife Edge**. **Rear Heel Scoop Kicks** might be thought of as the reverse motion of the **Front Snap Ball**. So-called circular kicks such as the **Inside or**

Outside Full Moon Kick are merely an elongated version of the **Front Snap Ball Master Key Kick** with circular rotation of the knee and hip joint. The **Master Key FOR Kicking** would be the uplifted knee. Figure 22 assesses the Master Key Kick known as the Front Snap Kick. Figure 22 illustrates both the **Front Snap Ball Kick** and **Front Thrust Kick** from initiation to full extension, while the final and larger picture in the series shows the **Front Thrust Kick** variant of the **Master Key** with **Forward Pelvic Tilt** and **Full Joint Lockout** at **Full Extension** utilized for penetration and to bring the hip into play in the generation of power.

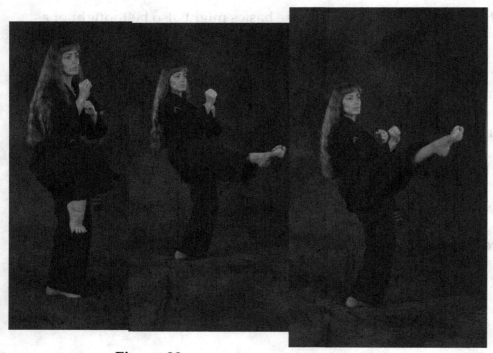

Figure 22

The **Chop Kick** is yet another **Master Key Basic** illustrated in Figures 23 and 24. This basic is executed in a unique fashion in the modern American Wu Shen Pai Kenpo system. The Chop Kick is executed as an off angle Front Snap

Kick. This far more direct method of execution has a number of advantages. First, it is more economical in terms of motion. When delivered at the forty-five degree angle as illustrated, it is the most direct line of motion to the target from the point of origin. It might truly be said that if there is a mortal sin in Kenpo, it is found in the lack of economy of motion. Second, this form of the Roundhouse Kick is harder to block than the conventional delivery of the Roundhouse Kick which is a thrust kick, at a 90 Degree Angle relative to the opponent. Third, the kick comes in just under the opponent's Zones of Obscurity, making it more difficult to spot when incoming. Fourth, and perhaps most important, this method of execution allows for the delivery of kicks to the opponent's upper height zones without a great deal of flexibility training since it does not employ the hamstring muscle actively in its execution. Figure 23 shows the cocked position of the Chop Kick from a variety of angles.

Figure 23

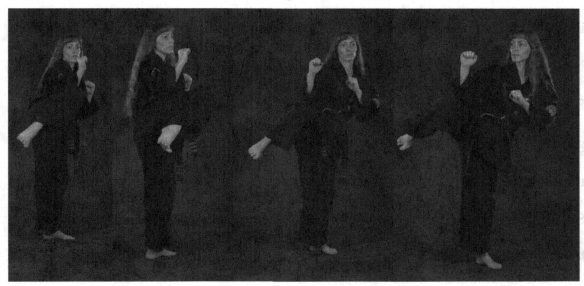

Figure 24 shows the Chop Kick from inception to full execution from the frontal angle. As with all kicks, snapping differs quite significantly from thrusting in terms of hip rotation and lock out at full extension. The Chop Kick

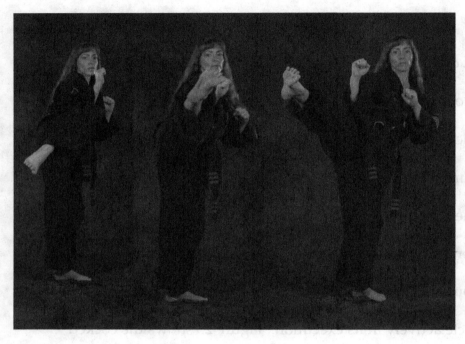

does not rotate the hips over for maximum penetration through the target. It uses Whip as a Master Key Method of Execution.

Figure 24

The **Roundhouse Kick**, or the thrusting variant of the **Chop Kick**, is illustrated in figure 25. When the **Roundhouse Kick** is executed in Wu Shen Pai, it might be described as a Chop Kick with Thrust as the Master Key method of Execution, the hips rotate through and the leg and foot are parallel to the ground. This enables the foot to penetrate more deeply into the target while still maintaining the **Proper Body Alignment** through the use of the **Angle of Scaption** with the hips. The joints in a Thrusting Roundhouse Kick reach full lock out which is held for seconds in the execution of the basic during impact.

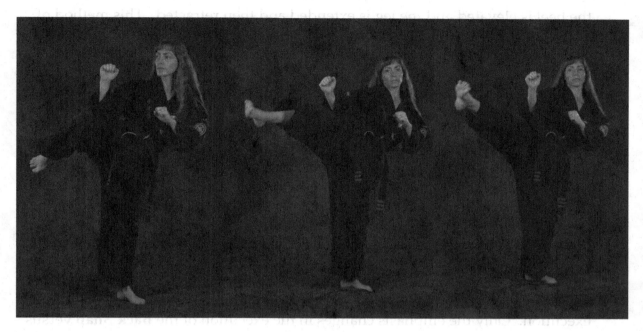

Figure 25

The Back Kick in Wu Shen Pai Kenpo has two variants, the Back Thrust and the Back Snap Kick.

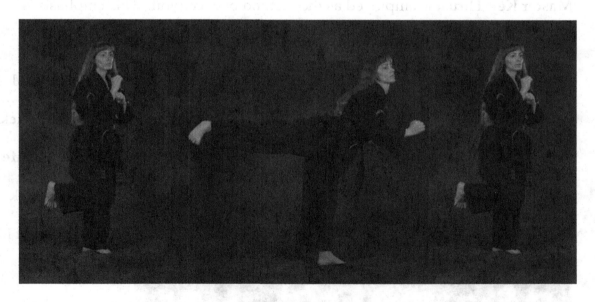

Figure 26

Figure 26 illustrates the proper execution of a **Back Snap Kick**. This basic is yet another **Master Key Basic**. In executing the **Master Key Back Snap Kick**, the heel is elevated and the leg is extended and then retracted. This method of execution is the most direct to the target. Notice that the knee is not raised to the front first since this would violate the **Principle of Economy of Motion**. Once again, the basic fails to telegraph intent and is executed in such a way that it moves in under the opponent's **Zones of Obscurity**. This method executing the Back Snap Kick also has the merit of creating spinal alignment, thus placing the body mass behind the impact force of the kick. This kick does not change physically when executed with the **Master Key Thrust** as its method of execution. Only the emphasis changes in the execution of the **Back Snap** versus the **Back Thrust**. The emphasis is placed on the retraction in the **Back Snap Kick** while the emphasis shifts to the extension of the kick into the target when the **Master Key Thrust** is employed as the method of execution. This emphasis is shifted since joint lock out occurs in this kick, as in other thrusting kicks.

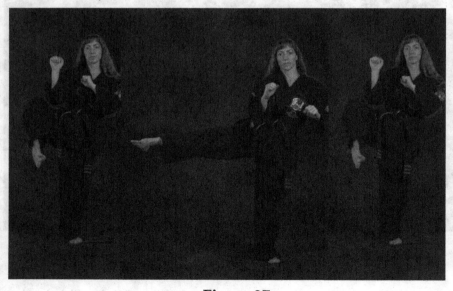

The final **Master Key Kick** is the **Side Knife Edge**. This kick is shown at left in Figure 27. As illustrated, the leg is cocked into

Figure 27

the **Master Key for Kicking** and then fired to the side or the front and immediately retracted. The striking surface of the foot is the knife-edge and heel of the foot. The difference between the **Side Knife Edge** where **Whip** is the **Master Key Method of Execution** and the **Side Thrust Kick** where **Thrust** is the **Master Key Method of Execution** lies in the rotation of the hips and the flexion and lock out of the joints at full extension. The hips ideally rotate such that the toes point slightly downward and the striking surface is the heel and edge of the foot. The execution of the Side Thrust Kick is illustrated below in Figure 28.

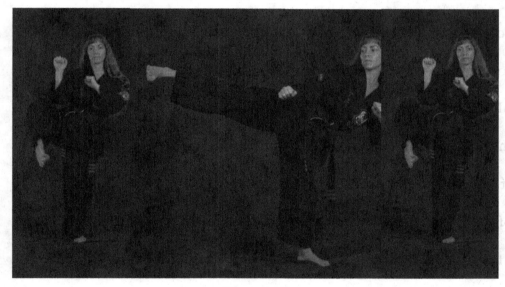

Figure 28

Master Key Basics – Foot Maneuvers

The **Master Key Foot Maneuvers** are the **Push Drag** and the **Pull Drag**. All other foot maneuvers are variants of these. Some would assert that a Master Key known as "launch" exists. This view stems from a misunderstanding of Master Key Basics and their role in the proper execution of the physical constituents of motion. Launch is not a Master Key of any sort, but is a force

derived from the proper, forceful execution of Master Key Basics such as a Push

Drag or other foot maneuver.

The Significance of Master Key Basics

The importance of Master Keys lies in the **process of training for mastery**

of the art and for understanding the art cannot be minimized. The importance of

Master Key Basics is simple. They can be re-defined to deal effectively with a

multitude of dilemmas in either an offensive or defensive fashion. They can be,

once understood in this way, utilized to cut the training time for mastery of the

art dramatically. For example, by mastering the concept of the Inward Block, I

also master the concept of the Inward Back Knuckle Rake. To use another

illustration, If I understand the concept of the Upward Block, I also understand

the concept of the Upward Forearm Strike since the knowledge of one leads

invariably to the mastery of both. The concepts of the Inward and Upward Block

are merely the defensive application of the motion, while the concepts of the

Upward Forearm Strike and the Inward Back Knuckle Rake are the offensive

applications. There are few great differences between the Inward Block and the

Back Knuckle Rake. Depth of Penetration is one such difference. Another is

intent. Was it your intention to block or strike? With respect to the Upward

Forearm Strike and the Upward Block, some physical differences exist, such as

the height of the strike or physical motion in addition to depth of penetration and intent. Some Master Key Basics such as the Straight Thrust Punch when subject to scrutiny will be found identical to other basics such as the Straight Finger Thrust. The only difference between these two basics being the deployment of different natural weapons to different targets, although both basics employ the same **Master Key Method of Execution**, which is a **Thrusting Master Key Method of Execution.**

Truly understanding Master Keys in the arena of kicking has profound importance in two senses. First, by understanding the **Primary** and **Secondary Master Keys For Kicking** and the **Master Key Kicks**, we might make our kicking applications more efficient. For example, we might better understand the efficient generation of, and the use of, compound motion. This is where multiple impressions are made upon an opponent utilizing a single movement.

Second, In terms of our training, the importance of **Master Key Basics** is profound. They enable us to truly focus our training efforts on a limited number of skill sub-sets which in turn lead to mastery of a broader series of skill sets. By thus employing our understanding of Master Keys in all their applications, we will be able to cut the training time necessary for the mastery of the art to a fraction of what it may have been previously. To master, for example, 365 kicks would require the constant drill of each of them. In utilizing our understanding of **Master Key Kicks**, we might drill a limited number of kicks to a finer degree of skill and hence master the skill sets necessary to be able to execute with minor alteration the entire set of kicks. By saving time in our training, we train more intelligently. More to the point, this enables us to more broadly focus on all aspects of the art, rather than having to specialize in the development of kicking skills, aiding us in our mastery of these skills and in the art as a whole.

Whether we are employing basics with the hand and arm, or with the foot and leg, proper utilization and understanding of the Master Key Basics in our training leads to profound shortcuts in the attainment of greater efficiency and skill in our quest for self-mastery. For this reason alone, they deserve proper scrutiny and appreciation.

Chapter Two: *Physical Constituents of Power and the Mental Master Keys: Physiological Engagement in the Master Key Stances*

The most fundamental of **Master Key Basics** is **the Neutral Bow and Arrow Stance**, or the Neutral Bow for short. This is so since what we might term **Physiological Engagement** is achieved with a proper understanding and application of this Master Key Basic. **Physiological Engagement** is the most foundational level at which we apply the physical principles of power. This term is simply, the steadying or securing of the body such that when impact is made against a target there is stabilization of the weapon and hence greater infliction of damage upon, or penetration into, the target. To put this in other terms, it is our kicking the heavy bag in such a way that the bag moves and we do not. We might liken our body mechanics without Physiological Engagement to being like engaging in a fight while on roller skates. Making contact which serves to damage the attacker in such circumstances is truly unlikely. Compare this with being back on our own two feet once again, and one can readily appreciate the role which the **Stabilization of our Base** plays in ensuring solid execution of our movements, whether they may be offensive or defensive. **Physiological Engagement** primarily refers to the position of the ball and socket joints of the body, our hips and shoulders, such that they are locked in place to provide a brace for hand strikes. This is accomplished by positioning the hips and shoulders in such a way, relative to the opponent, that such stability is achieved.

This position is arrived at for the hips by pointing the feet toward the forty-five degree angle with the heels of the feet pressed out as in the illustration. See figure 32 and note the position of the feet at a 45 Degree angle relative to the 12 o'clock position.

The impact upon hitting power is readily apparent. We can even compare the hitting power in a neutral bow with physiological engagement to that achieved with the lead foot pointed forward, for example. This principle, coupled with forward projection, is essential for dynamic hitting power. This is, however, only a partial view of how vital this principle might be. When

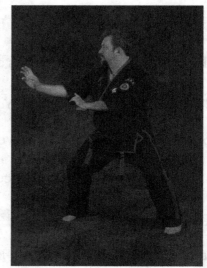

Figure 29

we look at Physiological Engagement with the hands and arms, we might better appreciate the impact which this principle has upon building power in our strikes. Both the shoulder and the hip joints function as ball and socket joints. When set to the forty-five degree angle, in relation to the target, the arms move faster in their natural range of motion. This holds true since the muscles that are in opposition at other angles function to pull harmoniously at this angle. The arms, like the hips, are more stable when set at the 45 Degree angle in relation to the target than at any other. This is true since the arms, when the body is placed in the 45 Degree Angle relative the opponent, operate on the **Angle of Scaption**. Also known as "the Groove" in Anatomy and Physiology, it is the angle at which the arm operates most efficiently since **Gravitational Fall** comes into play and the muscles of the arm and shoulder are not in opposition. This enhances the natural muscular speed of the arm in action. One example for this stability, and for the enhanced action of the hand and arm within the **Angle of Scaption** might be discovered in the technique known in American Wu Shen Pai Kenpo

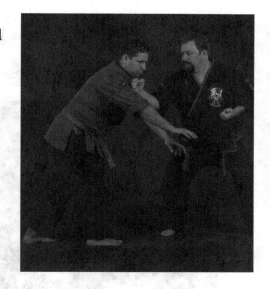

Figure 30

as Alternating Maces. On the initial movement for this technique, the 45 Degree angle might be employed in blocking utilizing the principle of **Pin Pointing**. The tremendous stability of this position actually impedes the forward momentum of the opponent pushing forward. Needless to say, when this angle is employed offensively, it is equally effective. The first move of Alternating Maces is illustrated in **Figure 30.**

What is truly significant in our understanding of **Physiological Engagement** as it pertains to self-defense is how our body stability, or **Solidification of our Base**, is tremendously enhanced through the use of a forty-five degree **Angle of Execution** relative to the opponent. This occurs because of the "lock down" of the ball and socket joint at this angle, relative to the opponent. Note the **Stabilization** and **Solidification of the Base** that is enhanced as a result of the proper use of angles of Engagement. Another example of the tremendous stability that is obtained through **Physiological Engagement** of the

Neutral Bow is found in the Wu Shen Pai technique Mace of Aggression. The

offensive application of these principles is shown below in Figure 31.

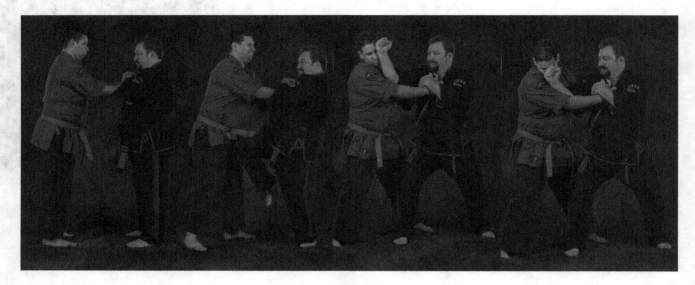

Figure 31

One of the more commonly understood principles expressed in the second

move of the Yellow Belt technique Alternating Maces is that of the **Bracing**

Angle. This occurs as the result of the brace which the locking out of the left leg

provides to afford greater stability and power to the left hand punch delivered

with the rotation of the body forward into a Forward Bow and Arrow stance or

Forward Bow. The leg serves to brace the entire upper body in this

circumstance, and in all like circumstances, ensuring the impact force of the left

hand punch. Less commonly understood is the element of **Physiological**

Engagement which accompanies the **Bracing Angle** of the left leg in a right

Neutral Bow. This element occurs on the right side of the body simultaneously

with the bracing angle. This principle of **Physiological Engagement** is known as

Forward Projection. Both the principle of the **Bracing Angle** and the principle of **Forward Projection** as part of **Physiological Engagement** are illustrated in Figure 32 from various angles. Note the turned in front foot, the locked out rear knee, the direct forward angle of the toes of the rear foot and the vertical line of the shin. All of these principles expressed in this illustration of the Forward Bow and Arrow stance are integral to the physical expression of the principles of Bracing Angle and Forward Projection.

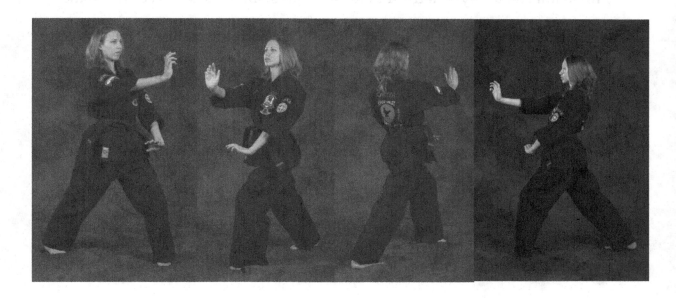

Figure 32

Forward Projection is the projection forward of body mass which, when done without violating any other principles and concepts such as **Proper Body Alignment**, further empowers the strike through the use of Back Up Mass. This principle is the result of the manipulation of the three zones of defense in such a way that stability is maximized for the lead leg. This principle establishes tremendous **Forward Stability**. The stability in the position of a **Forward Bow and Arrow Stance** is due both to **Forward Projection** and the **Bracing Angle.** The concept of the **Bracing Angle** is employed by turning the rear foot completely forward, toes straight ahead with the rear knee locked out. Forward Projection is achieved by turning the toes of the front foot to the forty-five degree angle and pushing the knee forward This **Bracing Angle** coupled with **Forward Projection** creates **Symmetrical Stability**. This stability is achieved due to the alignment of the skeletal structure, allowing the body's weight and mass to rest on the skeletal structure for support. This serves to free up the musculature of the body for movement, since it is no longer responsible for the support of the body mass. For example, in the illustration below, the knee rests over the toes. This is the sure sign that **Forward Projection** has been achieved. By doing this, immovable structural stability is established for rear hand, or lead hand, strikes in such techniques as Alternating Maces.

Another aspect of forward projection which is evident in this stance as utilized in the technique Alternating Maces has to do with a concept derived from forward projection known as forward pelvic tilt. This concept not only serves to check the groin from direct attack from in front and behind, it also locks down the hips and further accentuates the structural stability of the forward bow and arrow stance. Moreover, as has been previously asserted, when we employ forward projection, we also place the lead knee over the lead toes. This creates an almost immovable structural stability which is based on the proper alignment of the skeletal structure of the hips, knees, thighs, and spinal column of the human body. The skeletal structure in the natural movement of American Kenpo performs its function of supporting the body weight, leaving the muscles free to perform their given function of positioning and moving the body.

Forward projection might be understood statically and dynamically. When we utilize it dynamically, it is not so much that we seek stability in defensive settings, or in employing a defensive offense. It is rather that we employ our forward motion in a form of "**Ballistic Projection**" such that our body mass and skeletal structure more serve as a backup mass for the strikes or series of strikes performed in this manner. **Forward Ballistic Projection** when utilized in conjunction with a launching action of any sort create **Horizontal Momentum** in a forward direction. This may be readily converted to **Rotational Momentum**. The maximum impact is possible, however, only at the forty five degree angle since any power involved in a strike rapidly dissipates after that point.

Both **Forward Projection** and **Physiological Engagement**, as principles, are perceived from a relative perspective which serves to reinforce for us the importance of a **Master Key Basic,** the **Neutral Bow**. Put in more "Master Key" terms, the value of the Neutral Bow is perhaps best understood as being the means through which the body is placed into a 45 Degree **Angle of Alignment** relative to the opponent at all times. Without the **Proper Body Attitude**, it is impossible to achieve what we term in Kenpo as "**Proper Body Alignment**".

Proper Attitude is the appropriate employment of **Physiological Engagement** and **Forward Projection** obtained through the maintenance of a neutral position in which we place the body behind the action initiated thus achieving **Proper Body Alignment**. **Proper Attitude** is achieved when we maintain proper toe-heel alignment in our **Neutral Bow**. Taken together with the various mechanical elements in the dynamics of body motion maximum efficiency is achieved through the summation of principles so that Back Up Mass is attained.

When we consider the importance of the physical constituents of power such as the **Bracing Angle** and **Forward Projection** to our **Physiological Engagement**, one important realization emerges which the serious long-term student of the art ultimately comes to appreciate is the importance of stance work. Stances are the most essential foundations of the art and the basis of any increased power realized. More specifically, effective and proper stance work holds the key to Proper Body Alignment. Our Proper Body Alignment is defined not only in terms of our body position relative to the opponent. This Mr. Parker aptly termed "**position**" and is considered it so he vital that it occupied a place as one of Mr. Parker's so-called "**Eight Considerations**" for attack and defense. It is necessary to view position as central to the context of **Three-Dimensional Hitting**, environment, and physiological engagement in order to fully appreciate these sets of relationships.

Proper Body Attitude, or the maintenance of the proper 45 Degree angle for the hips and shoulders relative to the opponent, becomes critical when we understand the relationship that this angle has with respect to the execution of hand and arm movements along the Angle of Scaption. The **Angle of Scaption** so essential to speed, and hence to power, is lost without a proper 45 Degree angle in relation to the target. We also lose **Proper Body Alignment** when our attitude is incorrect with respect to the opponent's body. Taken together this may reduce our potential power by as much as fifty or sixty percent. This is Proper Body Attitude, or the attitude of the body vis a vis the opponent, viewed from the static perspective. From the dynamic perspective, it is impossible to obtain great power once we pass the forty-five degree angle line or path or execution with our motion. The apex of the circle, in other words, is our moment of greatest impact power. Figure 33 pictures the principle of the Angle of Scaption applied to the other ball and socket joint of the body, the hips.

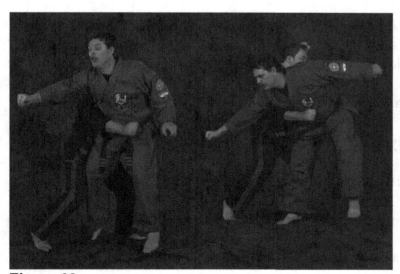

Figure 33

It is important to understand that these principles in Wu Shen Pai Kenpo are not merely examined in the abstract. The entire system was conceived as a vehicle to discover the underlying truths inherent in the concepts and principles of motion. It is this which defines the essence of Wu Shen Pai Kenpo. Unlike other arts, American Wu Shen Pai Kenpo techniques, Forms, and Sets exist as models for the various principles and concepts of motion. Eventually the importance of technique memorization pales beside the mastery of formulation in harmony with these concepts and principles of motion. At this phase of understanding, the various techniques, forms, and sets are useful only to guide other practitioners to this same level of understanding with respect to motion.

Physiological Factors of Engagement

In order to arrive at any understanding of the importance of the Angle of Scaption, it is essential to look at the bio-mechanical constituents and physiological effects of the employment of the Angle of Scaption. It is important to understand that the angle of scaption functions with both sets of ball and socket joints in the body. In the hips, the Angle of Scaption is utilized to stabilize the arms and place the body behind the action of the strike. When a kick is the weapon of choice, placing the hips on the Angle of Scaption has the effect of placing the body mass behind the action. In both instances, the Angle of Scaption, whether used as a bracing angle, or to effect back up mass, increases the power of the strike. This is how we arrive at the term "Proper Body

Alignment". A body alignment which is improper would be one which moves the hips, the shoulders, or both ball and socket joints off the angle of scaption. The resulting decrease in power is rooted in the loss of back up mass and, when movement is attempted, body momentum. When standing in place, the positioning of the heels in the stance is of critical importance. When Physiological Engagement is lost, then the hips are no longer locked down with the resulting decrease in power due to loss of stability. The body functions, under these circumstances at rest, as a platform for the striking weapon. Forward projection is the act of projecting forward the body mass in potential movement in such a fashion that back up mass is the result while the body is at rest. Forward projection while the body is in motion is the act of projecting the body mass, or generating body momentum, forward in such a way that back up mass is realized ballistically in terms of potential energy moving into kinetic energy. As we can see, the notions of physiological engagement, the angle of scaption, proper body alignment, attitude, back up mass, and body momentum are so intertwined that in order to maximize power, and hence efficiency, all of these physiological constituents to power must be working together in such harmony that the loss of any one of them seriously impedes the development of power in our strikes or kicks. To simplify this explanation, if we position our body in such a way as to obtain proper body alignment, then we obtain all of these physical constituents of power. In Figure 34, the notion of Macro and Micro Body alignment is explored. **Macro Body Alignment is the presence of Proper Body**

Alignment in all its components. **Macro Body Alignment** exists when both the upper and lower body are behind the action or movement performed. **Micro Body Alignment** is the presence of **Proper Body Alignment** in its various parts. **Micro Body Alignment**, when it exists in all the component parts of a movement, result in **Macro Body Alignment**. In the inset illustration at right, it is possible to observe the **Micro Alignment** of the fist, hand, and arm. The fore knuckles are aligned with the wrist which is aligned with the forearm and the shoulder. In Figure 34, the left illustration shows **Macro Body Alignment** which is the combination of **Forward Projection**, a **Bracing Angle**, and Forward Pelvic Tilt which is enabled by the proper foot positioning and proper stance work. Contributing to **Macro Body Alignment** is proper posture, which should be ramrod straight, enabling the full utilization of **Rotational Momentum**. When we achieve Macro Body Alignment, we might be said to be fully engaged physiologically. This arises from our **Summation of Forces**, which come into alignment through the achievement of **Macro Body Alignment**.

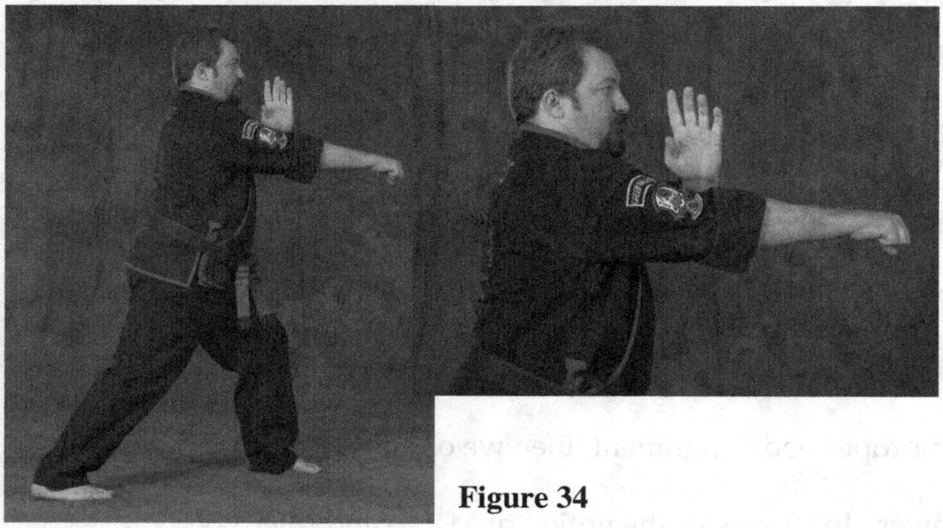

Figure 34

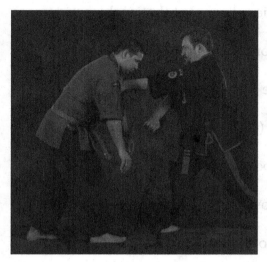

Another factor to consider is lower case motion when looking at macro and micro body alignment. Figure 35 shows the second movement in the Wu Shen Pai technique Alternating Maces. This movement entails both macro and micro body alignment in the lower case.

Figure 35

The Power Equation and its Purpose

Physical or bodily alignment is a sufficient and necessary condition for the achievement of our maximum power potential. However, it is not the only condition which must be present. There is the factor of physical speed, for example. **Proper Body Alignment** allows us to maximize our **Back Up Mass**, or as it is termed in physics, mass. Mass and speed are related to the various forms of momentum in creating maximum power for minimum effort, or maximum efficiency. One method of understanding the relationship between the various factors that go into generating power is the **Master Key Concept** of the **Power Equation**.

The **Power Equation** is one of **the MASTER KEY CONCEPTS** of American Kenpo, or simply put, it is a foundational concept that enables us to more readily grasp relationship of various factors within the art. The Power Equation is expressed thus: ½ M $(V)^2$ = F where Mass if defined as M=[(rm)(hm)(vm)] PBA. Velocity is defined as (d) (r) (t) = V. This equation expresses the principle relationships between power and speed, a great controversy in American Kenpo. For this purpose it is possible to use a simple physics equation for calculating force which more effectively explores the relationship between speed and power by inserting values, however arbitrary, into the equation. For illustration purposes let us assert that there are both 2 units of Mass and 2 units of Velocity.

Then:	Doubling the values for Mass:	Doubling the values for Velocity:
½ M $(V)^2$=F	½ M $(V)^2$=F	½ M $(V)^2$=F
½ $(2)(2)^2$=F	½ $(4)(2)^2$=F	½ $(2)(4)^2$=F
(1)(4)=F	(2)(4)=F	(1)(16)=F
F=4	F=8	F=16

If we examine the series of equations above, the implications for the relationship of speed to power are quite clear. It is indisputable that by doubling speed, power is quadrupled while a commensurate increase in Mass with the

62

variable of speed held as a constant results only in doubling the power of the strike. Mr. Parker stated that he was not afraid of guns, it was the bullets that he feared. If a bullet were to be handheld and thrown toward an opponent, then it is safe to state that it would hold no terror. If, however, we insert that bullet into a magazine and then into a pistol, the respect for the bullet as a weapon is greatly magnified. This is true since the muzzle velocity of the bullet, its speed, has increased so as to allow it to penetrate our body. In this illustration, the mass of the bullet is self contained and the muzzle velocity would be all important in defining power to penetrate. In this circumstance, speed IS power.

With the human body, it is also important to have Mass. Let us examine that relationship momentarily. If we take the same equation and decrease Proper Body Alignment, then it serves to decrease our Mass. This is illustrated in the second equation. The last equation shows the impact of losing Proper Body Alignment so much so that we lose all Mass.

Then:	Decreasing our Mass:	
$\frac{1}{2} M (V)^2 = F$	$\frac{1}{2} M (V)^2 = F$	$\frac{1}{2} M (V)^2 = F$
$\frac{1}{2} (2)(2)^2 = F$	$\frac{1}{2} (1)(2)^2 = F$	$\frac{1}{2} (0)(4)^2 = F$
$(1)(4) = F$	$(1/2)(4) = F$	$(0)(4) = F$
$F = 4$	$F = 2$	$F = 0$

Within the last equation for mass, Proper Body Alignment, an essential element of the equation is lost. We can see that this drops the force obtained to zero. We can also see from this relationship that Proper Body Alignment is both a necessary and sufficient condition for power. What this means is that no mass is possible without Proper Body Alignment and consequently no power. All of these formulas, in the abstract, allow us to assess relationships. Now that we have assessed the relative relationships of mass and speed to each other, it is important to define the dynamics of the relationships between the various elements of mass as they pertain to the art of Wu Shen Pai Kenpo. Mass, in the context of physics and for our purposes as Kenpoists, references what is termed Back Up Mass defined through a portion of the so-called "Power equation". This equation was a formula which was adapted from physics to explain the relationship which the various elements of mass hold to one another. As we recall, the power equation as a whole expressed relationships between speed and mass: $\sum \frac{1}{2} (M) (V)^2$ = Force.

Mass, in this equation is expressed where $M = \sum [(rm) (vm) (hm)]$ PBA. Or stated more succinctly, where **mass is the sum of rotational momentum, horizontal momentum, and vertical momentum, multiplied by Proper Body Alignment.** The summed and hence exponential values of **Horizontal Momentum, Vertical Momentum, and Rotational Momentum** are what form the basis for **Back Up Mass** or more simply mass. We in American Kenpo use the term "Back Up Mass" as the substitute for the more common usage of the term "mass" utilized in physics. This implies the usage of the mass. It is truly used for "back up" in the execution of the strike or kick employed.

Horizontal Momentum is obtained through Shuffling or employing foot maneuvers to achieve greater impact in our strikes by placing the body weight behind the horizontal motion of our strikes. Another way to describe this method of achieving horizontal momentum is to say that we launch horizontally. Vertical Momentum is obtained through Drop by marrying gravity to our blow. By doing this we further enhance the value of the strike. Rotational Momentum is obtained through rotation of the hips. This serves to enhance the power of the strike through either centrifugal force or through direct impact obtained through direct body rotation. We can also say that Counter Body Rotation would give us power in this way. Counter Body Rotation is when the hips rotate in the opposite direction from that of the strike. This serves to increase the speed of the limb through the process of tightening the fulcrum and results in the execution of the master key whip, through a mechanism that strongly resembles the effect of cracking a bull whip.

What holds further significance with respect to these forms of obtaining power through body mechanics is that they relate to manipulation of the three Zones of Defense. These are Zones of Height, Zones of Width, and Zones of Depth. When employing Rotational Momentum, for example, we manipulate our Zones of Width. Height Zones are manipulated to achieve drop and hence gravitational marriage, while Depth Zones are manipulated when we utilize shuffle to achieve **Horizontal Momentum**. The achievement of these forces summated thus might be construed as being "**Three Dimensional Hitting**." This term would hold true since all three dimensions are being employed to maximum effect in the strike. This conception of power hitting is markedly different from that found in classical martial arts. The following illustration shows the Wu Shen Pai Kenpo self defense technique known as Sword and Hammer performed with three dimensions in the strikes. It is possible to execute the technique with one or two dimensions involved in the strikes. To execute the technique with only one dimension, that of depth, involved in the strike, it is necessary only to step straight out into horse stance and execute the first move. This limits the range of motion and seriously retards both penetration and power. To strike with both depth and height in the Hand Sword, it is necessary merely to drop more deeply into the horse stance. To strike with all three dimensions, height, width, and depth, it is necessary to step out into a Neutral Bow stance with the initial Hand Sword as pictured in Figure 36. Experimentation will show that greater power is obtained when all three dimensions are employed in striking.

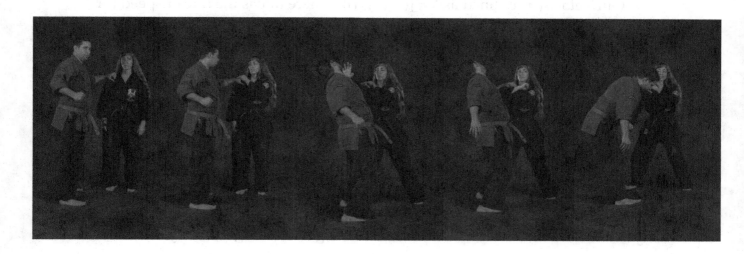

Figure 36

To review, our understanding of mass when expressed mathematically is

M = Σ [(RM) (VM) (HM)] PE. This much is somewhat standard fare in high

school physics courses across America. **Proper Body Alignment**, a term which

we apply specifically to Wu Shen Pai Kenpo, is in turn defined as the subset of

Physiological Engagement multiplied by the forward projection of our weight,

the bracing angles employed, and both micro and macro body alignment. Stated

mathematically, **Proper Body Alignment** is expressed as PE = [(fp) (ba) (pba)].

Where fp = Forward Projection, ba = Bracing Angle, and pba = Proper Body

Alignment. Proper Body Alignment is properly understood as PBA = Σ[(Micro

Body Alignment) (Macro Body Alignment)] where PBA = Proper Body

Alignment is the sum of the multiplicative properties of Micro Body Alignment,

and Macro Body Alignment. These factors are aided by our able employment of

our zones of offense.

Our velocity is defined as $V = [(r)(d)(t)]^2$ where rate is the rate of speed (or physical speed of our motion), distance is the distance to the target and time is the time it takes us to travel to the target at our constant speed. This is squared. Put another way, our velocity is defined in terms of our physical speed, which is enhanced by increasing our speed of execution to the main target through a principle termed "elastic recoil", or by rounding off corners and elongating circles which lead us to cut the distance to the target. Most significantly, for Wu Shen Pai Kenpo, there is a third method of increasing speed which is often overlooked. This method is inherent in such principles as meeting force and entails taking full advantage of the opponent's anticipated response to our various strikes such that he (or she) will actually move physically toward the strike itself. By employing this principle, the opponent actually aids us by moving toward us thus decreasing the distance to target.

There are those who would argue perhaps that an analysis of this sort has no place in the martial arts. I would hold that, to the contrary, such an analysis enables us to rely on evidence in order to reach a conclusion about how we generate power and the relationship between and among variables. This does not replace the crucible of hard won knowledge through training, it merely eliminates superstition and prejudice in our understanding of these variables.

Chapter Three: Master Key Techniques

No discussion of Master Keys would be complete without, in some sense, assessing Master Key Techniques. For our purposes, we will look at this category of Master Keys as being divided into Primary and Secondary Master Key Techniques. Primary Master Key Techniques consist of the twelve Yellow Belt Techniques taught within the Wu Shen Pai system of Kenpo. Then there are Nine Secondary Master Key Techniques sprinkled throughout the Orange, Purple, and Blue Belt levels of American Wu Shen Pai Kenpo. When I reference the levels of material in the system, it is perhaps important to note that there is significant difference of opinion as to how the base curriculum should be taught, and at what point various aspects of it should be taught. There is also broad disagreement as to the value and purpose of extensions taught beyond the base system. For our purposes, when referencing levels of material taught, it will be done within the framework of the so-called "24 system" of techniques within American Wu Shen Pai Kenpo. This reference point, for those unfamiliar with it, may be found in the appendix.

The "Master Key" definition of master keys holds that they are a single move or series of moves that provide the solutions to a multitude of predicaments. We have already examined how basics might fit this definition. In this chapter, we will delve further into the meaning and significance of **Master Key Techniques**. In categorizing the various Master Key Techniques, it may be useful to view them as either Primary or Secondary in nature. There are

techniques which, to use a language analogy, might be construed as "root

words" of sorts for the language of motion which we are studying within Wu

Shen Pai Kenpo. For that matter, the concept of having root words of motion

might be found within a number of other martial disciplines as well. In Wu Shen

Pai Kenpo these roots of the study of motion are found within the Yellow Belt

syllabus. It is the techniques found within this level of study that are categorized

as Primary Master Key Techniques.

  Primary Master Key Techniques teach concepts which are or should be

nearly axiomatic in every movement. These concepts and principles include

Utilization of Three Dimensional Hitting, Proper Body Alignment, Narrowing

Targets, Creating Distance, Stabilization of the Base, Solidification of the Base,

Mastery of the Four Methods of Execution, Utilizing the Angle of Scaption or

the Master Key Movements. These Primary Master Key Techniques also teach

the utilization of different points on the circle when the motion of the first moves

from the first five Yellow Belt Techniques are examined. This is yet another way

of looking at the Master Key Movement as it is taught in the Primary Master Key

Techniques. Both **Primary** and **Secondary Master Key Techniques** entail the

study of the **Master Key Patterns.** The Primary Master Key Techniques also

teach concepts related to **Body Contouring** such as **Angle Matching,**

Complimentary Angle, and **Fitting**. **Physiological Engagement, Bracing Angle,**

and **Forward Projection** are also significant principles referenced within the

twelve Primary Master Key Techniques. It is, however, their ability to serve as an answer to a series of predicaments that make the **Master Key Technique** truly "Master Key". It is their status as a true "root word" of motion that serves to denote their **Primary** status within the system. I reference twelve rather than ten since the Wu Shen Pai syllabus includes the techniques Aggressive Twins and Intellectual Departure.

In all fairness, it is significant to note that the twelve (or ten for that matter) Yellow Belt techniques are not included in any list of "Master Key Techniques" generated by anyone. However, it is also true that when the listing of Secondary Master Key Techniques was originally generated, the Yellow Belt curriculum was not even in existence, since the other techniques of the base system preceded it in time. Even a cursory examination of the Yellow Belt Techniques would disclose that they are in essence "root words" of the other techniques. Hence my designation of the Yellow Belt techniques as **"Primary Master Key Techniques"** while other techniques so listed are considered **"Secondary Master Key Techniques."** What is also significant about the **Primary Master Key Techniques**, aside from what has already been discussed, is their value as models for fundamental **Master Key Concepts** such as "With", teaching us defensive and offensive applications for the same basics which is also known as "Redefining Basics", and their status as "root words" which lead to mastery of more complex "words" of motion. In addition to their use in this fashion, the **Primary Master Key Techniques** also serve as models for the **Master**

Key Methods of Execution and other forms of Master Keys which are foundational in nature. In addition, **Primary Master Key Techniques** also model principles such as **Forward and Reverse Motion** and act as category completion for certain typologies of movements.

While **Primary Master Key Techniques** have to do with mastering fundamental concepts and principles of motion inherent in all martial arts, the **Secondary Master Key Techniques** have to do with the thorough exploration of grafting differing **Master Key Methods of Execution** and with Wu Shen Pai Kenpo's **Five Master Key Strategies**. These strategies form the basis for our understanding of how we might cope with all forms of attack. For example, with a weapon in flight, such as a punch, it is possible to go to the inside of the punch. Techniques such as Five Swords demonstrate this intent. It is also possible to go to the outside of the punch. Techniques such as Dance of Death demonstrate this strategy. It is also possible to go underneath the punch. Techniques such as Circles of Protection model this strategy, while techniques such as Raining Claw model the fourth strategy of going on top of the punch. It is also possible to go in between, as is demonstrated in the initial moves of the technique Taming the Mace. These five strategies hold true for all attacks. For example in the Category of Pushes, specifically two hand front pushes, there is an inside (Parting Wings), an outside (Alternating Maces), on top of (Hooking Wings), underneath (Thrusting Wedge), and in-between (Snaking Talon). Obviously there are instances in some attacks where one category or another might be omitted since it would be largely inappropriate in meeting the attack in question. For example, with single hand pushes, there is an inside (Triggered Salute), an outside (Glancing Salute), an on top of, underneath, or in between might not be altogether appropriate or most efficient in dealing with this form of attack. Master Key Strategies are discussed further in Chapter 9 where we address Mental Master Keys. **Secondary Master Key Techniques** still meet the definition of "providing a moves or series of moves which constitute the answer to a multitude of dilemmas. **Secondary Master Key Techniques** exist within another set of criteria. For **Secondary Master Key Techniques**, it is the fact that these techniques constitute more elaboration on the basic "root word" of motion which defines the status of these techniques as Secondary Master Key Techniques. Secondary Master Key Techniques are listed in the Second Degree Brown Belt Manual. These are **Thundering Hammers, Five Swords, Lone Kimono, Repeating Mace, Intellectual Departure, Locked Wing, Shielding Hammer, Thrusting Salute, Parting Wings, and Hooking Wings.**

It is my view that this list of Master Key Techniques should be re-assessed to include those techniques which are said to contain the "DNA" of the Wu Shen Pai Kenpo system. Such techniques constitute the lexicon of Secondary Master Key Techniques since they and they alone could be utilized to reconstruct most if not all of the key elements which form the Wu Shen Pai Kenpo system in the event that all the other techniques were deleted. Such techniques as **Flashing Wings, Flashing Mace, Circling the Horizon, Gathering Clouds, Crossing**

Talon, Clutching Feathers, Triggered Salute, Snapping Twigs, Leaping Crane, Shield and Sword, Shield and Mace, Clipping the Storm, Glancing Lance, Protecting Fans, Unfurling Crane, and Deceptive Panther fall within this definition of Secondary Master Key Techniques.

Master Keys, whether primary or secondary, are closely related to the conception of a **"Family Group"**. This term, like the term "Master Key", has been much discussed to little effect. Probably the only conceptualization of the **"Family Group"** which makes much sense is located within the notion of a **Positional Categorization** of the techniques. Techniques are indexed based on the initial positions of the right and left arms. These are termed the "mother" and "father" move. The initial point of origin for the right and left arms, coupled with the differing types of footwork possible in the initial moves of a sequence was the source of Family Grouping categorization. Movement in footwork was defined simply by such considerations as whether we step in or back, with the right or left foot. Blocking with the right or left hands while doing so become the key ideas in defining the various categories of Family Groups. Within this conceptualization of family groups, the mother moves are performed with the left hand while the right hand is associated with the father moves within family groups. Thus all male lineages follow with the right hand while all female lineages follow with the left. Sequential follow-up moves are viewed as brother or sister movements in a family grouping of techniques. Another way of thinking about this concept is to view it as an exploration of variables. Family

Groupings in this context become centered around a simple exploration of range, position, and maneuver based upon natural motion.

The Action Reaction Dilemma In Wu Shen Pai Kenpo

The value of Master Key techniques lies primarily in their usefulness in defusing the reaction time dilemma. Research suggests that when subjects are timed in their reaction to a given stimulus and have to respond with only one variable, then the response time is .33 of a second. When variables are added, then the reaction time goes up commensurate with the number of variables added. When a test subject is presented with a stimulus and two variables as the possible responses, then the stimulus-response time rises to .64 of a second. When the number of variables is increased to merely three, the response time is increased by one third to .96 of a second. When the variables grow, the response time grows by at least .33 of a second with each additional variable that the subject must consider in responding to the stimulus. This is known as Hick's Law. Hicks law is stated more formally in this fashion: *The time M(n) required to make a choice from a menu of n items rises with the log to the base two of n.*[1] Obviously this dilemma grows quite large when a system has thousands of possible responses. Even hundreds of possible responses would entail a reaction time so

---

[1] Hick, W. E. (1952). "On the Rate of Gain of Information." **Quarterly Journal of Experimental Psychology**, *4*, 11-26.

slow as to defeat any remote hope that the opponent's action might be defeated by your own reaction.

Hick's Law, started out as a paper written in 1952 and simply set up an equation, or a mathematical relationship between variables and reaction time. The mind takes time to decide between options. Stated in a more simplistic form, the time increases significantly with the greater number of variables or techniques. The terms "significantly" and "greater number" are the key unknowns in that equation. What is "significant" and how many are "greater" are the real questions when it comes to reaction time. Selection time gets compounded exponentially when a person has to select from several choices. Some research suggests that there is a doubling ratio associated with Hicks Law, or, for every two variables we must choose between, selection time doubles.

Research suggests that there is yet another form of reaction time known as SRT, or Simple Reaction Time. It takes an average of 150 milliseconds to decide to take a given course of action. That's considerably less than a quarter of a second, or 250 milliseconds. Time studies governing both SRT and Hick's Law are both given perspective when we consider that there are 1,000 milliseconds in one second. Based on the doubling rule with the common SRT average, then choosing between two choices would take 300 milliseconds. If we extend these calculations, three variables would require 600 milliseconds, four variables require 1 second and 200 milliseconds, five variables require 2 seconds and 400 milliseconds, while six variables take a 4 full seconds and 800 milliseconds. A martial artist could learn five different variables in response to a given stimulus. Doing so would mean 9 seconds and 600 milliseconds would pass before a choice would be made. A total shut down of response to a given stimulus would be the certain result if we go beyond this point in the variable selection process. Yet, this research is counter-intuitive. One begins to wonder how a football game can be played, how a jazz pianist functions, or how a bicyclist can pedal himself through a New York City rush hour. How does a boxer, who sees a spilt-second opening, select a jab, cross, hook, uppercut, or overhead blow. For that matter, how does a boxer decide to step back straight, to the right or to the left in an exchange? If he dares to throw combination punches how can he select them so quickly? Under this exponential increase rule, it would seem athletes would merely be capable of standing dumbfounded, as index cards of variables rolled through their heads in an attempt to select a correct course of action. Athletic performance studies would seem to call into question the so-called "doubling rule." We need not only look to athletes. How can a typist type so quickly? Consider all the possible selections on the keyboard of a computer. How can your read this typed essay? It would seem that the exponential rule of "doubling" with each variable would encounter serious empirical challenge. Hick provided in impetus for a massive body of research since 1952. Performance tests conducted since Hick's original study in 1952 suggests, whether the subject in question is the reaction time required to select among variables to successfully perform tasks such as drive a vehicle, fly an aircraft, play a given sport, or to select among variables in a psychology laboratory, an emerging picture of what Hick's original research teaches us is rapidly emerging. Larish and Stelmach, in a 1982 study, established that one could select from 20 complex options in 340 milliseconds, providing the complex choices have been previously trained.[2] One other study even had a reaction time of .03 milliseconds between two trained choices. Research by Mowbray and Rhoades, in 1959, suggests that after five months of training and 45,000 trials of practice that there was no difference between 4 choices and 2 choices in terms of reaction time at the end of that period.[3] According to a simple model, Reaction Time, or RT, is influenced by a several levels of processing. First, stimulus input and afferent conveyance to the brain. The second phase of response time is identification of the stimulus by the brain. The third phase of response or reaction time is central processing where a response is chosen and a motor response is established. Finally, the initiation of the action constituting the response or efferent conveyance is effected. This research, by Welford, suggests that Hick's Law is only valid when the reaction task is combined with the decision processes. Once stimulus response patterns are firmly established, deviations from Hick's Law will be observed. Welford's views with respect to

---

[2] Larish D., and Stelmach G.E., "Spatial Orientation of a Limb Using Egocentric Reference Points" *Perceptual Psychophysics*, July; 32(1)19-26, (1982).

[3] Mowbray,G.H. and Rhoades,M.V., "On the reduction of choice reaction times with practice", *Quarterly Journal of Experimental Psychology* (1959) 11:16-23.

speed are congruent with Wu Shen Pai Kenpo's perspective on speed.[4] There is

perceptual speed, or the rate at which there is the perception of a threat. Then,

there is **mental speed** in which a response is chosen and initiated. Finally, there

is **physical speed**, the actual physical execution of the movements in question.

Physical speed is not especially prone to development. We have what we have

in the way of genetics. The proportion of fast twitch muscles to slow twitch

muscles is reasonably set. Perceptual speed and mental speed are forms of speed

that may be trained, or developed.

What the research suggests in every instance is that there is no difference

found in reaction time at all when selecting from numerous, well-trained choices.

Well-trained alternatives or variable responses, are the key. It is not that Hick's

Law is found to be inoperative, it has merely become a limiting instance. New

learning methodologies have been created to increase SRT and overall reaction

times. One such training method, **Sequential Learning,** really reduces reaction

and selection time. Sequential Learning is the stringing of tasks together

working like connected notes in music. **Conceptual Learning** is another new

learning method that enhances the speed of reaction in variable selection. In

relation to survival training, this means a person first makes an either/or

conceptual decision such as the decision to "shoot/don't shoot," or, "move-

---

[4] Welford, A. T., "Choice Reaction Time: Basic Concepts." in A. T. Welford (Ed.),
Reaction Times. , Academic Press, New York, pp. 73-128: 1980.

in/move back" in combat handgun shooting. Rather than selecting from a series of hand blocks, in Conceptual Learning the martial artist does not waste milliseconds selecting specific blocks and footwork. Rather, the trained response in conceptual learning would be, for example, "Inward Block" and "step in" with one foot or the other. This limits the possible range of response patterns that is precisely the role played by Master Key fundamentals and by Master Key Techniques. The trained body then takes over, following paths learned from prior repetition training. Utilizing a response set of three deep is exactly what the early training in our Kenpo system advocates. Research has shown that four sequences may be pushing the limit for the non-athletic student, though there are those students who can handle more. Tailoring is a specific function of the technically proficient instructor since it would now be possible to teach the best suited responses to differing skill-levels and body shapes. Before martial artists and others bring up Hick's Law they need to know the rest of the science since the 1950s, that improved training really decreases reaction time, and not use Hick as an excuse to cage us down to one-step movement and motion that is primitive at best. Hick's Law has become a legacy of research. Hick's Legacy is really telling us to train regularly and more intelligently, not necessarily to learn less.

We might liken modern training methodologies to the training on a mental level that goes into the preparation for a championship match in chess. First, the chess master undergoes rigorous memorization of various opening combinations known to be commonly used. Second, the chess master plays "blitz" or speed chess. This helps the chess master develop an intuitive feel for position. It also aids the chess master in making decisions quickly and decisively. Obviously there are differences between physical training and mental preparation. It could be strongly asserted that the differences are less than the commonalities involved. For example, in Wu Shen Pai training, memorization of opening moves in chess might be akin to understanding the various types of Master Keys which is part of the standard training for all students in Wu Shen Pai Kenpo. One could also assert that the creative use of technique lines is very much like speed chess in that it requires the practitioner to develop an intuitive feel for position and to make decisions rapidly and decisively. There is also a role that contact plays in technique lines and in classes. The student who fails to prepare, prepares to fail. By actually making limited contact to all of the target areas employed in our techniques we actually learn about response to physical stimulus that is realistic, and not artificial. Those having contact made upon them, build resistance to the contact and the discomfort associated with it. There is at least the theoretical possibility that we might be struck by our opponent in a street fight. Should this occur, then the likelihood of our being mentally and emotionally disrupted so as to be taken out of the fight is greatly diminished if we practice with contact.

The modern Wu Shen Pai system meets the dilemma posed by Hicks Law in several ways. First, training is limited to a set parameter of fundamental skills that serve to branch out into wider ranging skill sets, based upon a foundation of Master Keys. Two, a thorough understanding of family groupings of techniques enable the Wu Shen Pai Kenpo practitioner to train a few select response patterns and, after assessment in the learning sequence, make the appropriate adjustment to the variables posed by the opponent. Master Key Techniques and the Master Key Movement make substantial contributions to this process.

Returning to our discussion of **Master Key Techniques**, we recall that when grouped together in family groups based upon categories of motion, the number of variables which we are forced to consider drop tremendously. We merely have to consider that there IS a weapon in flight and not necessarily whether that weapon is a right or a left. One example of this is found in a comparison of two Orange Belt Techniques, Thrusting Salute and Buckling Branch. In executing both techniques, we step off to 4:30 with the right foot and execute a left downward block. We follow up with a right front thrust kick and it is only then that the mechanics of the two techniques differ. Whether the opponent throws a right or left kick is irrelevant. We respond by stepping back with the right foot and executing a left downward block. Again, whether the opponent executes a right or left kick in his attack, we continue our response by executing a right rear leg front kick. If it is a right front kick attack, then the target is the groin / bladder and if it is a left front kick attack, then the kick is executed underneath to the groin. By this point in time, we have had the opportunity to survey and determine whether the opponent has in fact thrown a left or a right kicking attack. We finish the technique dependent upon which side the opponent has attacked with. If the opponent has thrown a front right thrust kicking attack, then we finish with a right stepping through heel palm to the jaw while if it is a left kicking attack, the finish is to the rear leg via a left side knife edge to the opponent's left knee. Another factor contributing to the importance of Master keys is the presence of the action-reaction dilemma in any martial art system as already discussed. The basis for this dilemma is the philosophical underpinnings within all of the Asian and non-Asian martial arts that limit the practitioner to defense rather than attack. The presence and use of Master Key Basics and Techniques within a system solves the reaction time crisis. With the Reaction Time Crisis in mind, it would seem apparent that those arts advocating large numbers of techniques taught for each type of attack have forgotten the all-critical element of reaction time in a street confrontation. Yet in opposition to this dilemma is the need for comprehensively treating the many possible self-defense scenarios that might arise so that the student is both forewarned and forearmed. Master Keys enable us to present one answer for a multitude of scenarios and are the basis for Family Groupings.

These Family Groupings of techniques and the Master Key Techniques are the Wu Shen Pai Kenpo answer to the "more is better" bug. There are, by most accounts, 19 of these groupings. They are based on categories of response based on an analysis of variables within the web of knowledge. Family Groupings are, by all accounts, highly subjective in composition. Yet, these Master Key

Techniques enable the defender to successfully evaluate a much simpler subset of variables and respond. For example, should the attacker throw a right step through punch, the response becomes a left Inward Block, stepping in. After this point, assessment occurs which enables the defender to choose between an upper height zone, middle height zone, or a lower height zone line of retaliation. Our choice is based upon whether the attacker is open in any one zone and not in the others and possibly determined by the opponent's position. To elaborate, should the opponent decide to throw a right punch and not step through, then the groin is open and the response is the Kenpo technique Dance of Death. Should the opponent step through with the punch and close the groin as a targeting option as the body rotates into position for the punch, the response becomes Thundering Hammers and the secondary follow up becomes a forearm strike to the ribs. Should the opponent cover the ribs and step through so as to close the groin as a target, then the secondary follow up becomes a ridge hand strike to the temporal lobe. These three techniques are the classic examples of a family group as Ed Parker taught them. What Dance of Death, Thundering Hammers, and Sleeper have in common is their membership a family group that is defined through the Step In Left Inward Block and a right hand point of origin at your right hip. They explore, together, the variables involved in Lower Height Zone, Middle Height Zone, and Upper Height Zone secondary follow up strikes.

Master Keys truly enable us, in other words, to present one solution that will suffice to answer a multitude of self-defense questions. Mr. Parker often likened master keys to the master keys of a hotel which, when employed, unlock **all** of the doors.

This would seem to be an apt analogy when we consider that by internalizing a limited number of basic responses to given attacks, we need only have the space in time to assess the variables which would require our adaptation in the street. As we previously discussed in our analogy to chess, great chess masters often spend months prior to a championship game reviewing opening strategy. This consists of studying the "accepted" or "strongest" moves with which to open the game. Somewhere in the middle game, a departure from known "lines" would occur which places the game on unique footing. The study of the multitude of possible opening lines is the search for advantage in the middle game. Thus, like a chess master armed for a championship match, we would have a basic glossary of "opening movements" so to speak which we would have internalized. Like that chess master, we would need only to memorize to a limited extent, then we would formulate based upon the requirements of the game, or the moves of the opponent. We would also have prepared for our street encounter by countless hours of work on a body that would enable us to evaluate the encounter from the three points of view. This type of preparation would also entail developing a feel for position. We would have mental and emotional clarity based on our contact oriented training which would have prepared us for the shock of combat.

Figure 37 illustrates two variables that may arise from a Step Through Inward Block. One is, of course, the middle zone secondary movement resulting from an inward forearm strike to the opponent's rib cage such as occurs when executing the Kenpo technique Thundering Hammers. The second is what results from a secondary retaliation to the groin with a reverse ridge hand such as occurs in the Kenpo technique Dance of Death. The third option would be to utilize an upper height zone secondary retaliation by executing the Kenpo technique Sleeper.

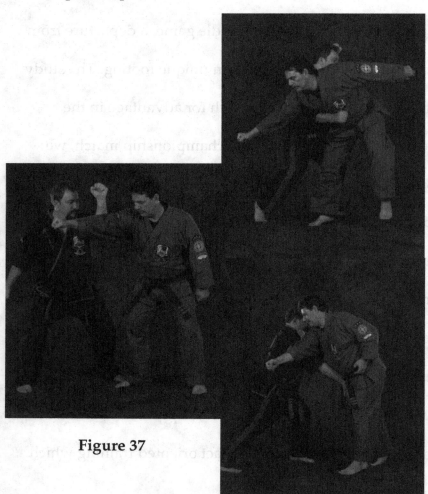

Figure 37

The Structure and Meaning of the Syllabus in Wu Shen Pai Kenpo

There is a structure and pattern to the syllabus in modern Wu Shen Pai Kenpo which, if altered, changes the meaning of the instructional content of the syllabus itself. There are **themes** within each belt which the techniques for each belt and the other elements of the instructional content of the syllabus communicate.

For example, **Orange Belt** has as its theme, the topic of **Rotational Momentum**. This theme includes both **Direct Body Rotation** and **Counter Body Rotation**. **Purple Belt** has as its theme the integration of skills in **Vertical and Horizontal Momentum** with the already established skills in **Rotational Momentum**. By this point in the student's career, he or she has learned how to generate power using all three dimensional zones. **Blue Belt** adds **Circularity of Motion** with our already established **Three Dimensional Hitting** capabilities. **Green Belt** has **Speed** and **Timing** as its theme. The themes of **3rd Degree Brown Belt** have to do with the transition from **Solid to Liquid States of Motion**, while the themes of **2nd Degree Brown Belt** have to do with the transition in our movement from **Liquid** to **Gaseous States of Motion**. **Paths of Motion** and **Lines of Motion** are explored as well at both of these levels.

When we begin to learn the 1st Degree Brown Belt extensions, this pattern repeats itself, concerning itself with the lower body instead of the upper body. For example, 1st Degree Brown Belt techniques, extensions of the Orange Belt, deal with the subject of lower body rotation as it is used to impact the various dimensional zones of the opponent. 1st Degree Black Belt techniques, extensions of the Purple Belt techniques, concern themselves with the utilization of all the dimensional zones of height, width, and depth in establishing **Horizontal, Vertical, and Rotational Momentum** impacting the opponent with the lower body. 2nd Degree Black Belt techniques, extensions of the Blue Belt techniques, actuate the circular motion of the lower body with the already established principles utilized to maximize power. 3rd Degree Black Belt techniques, extensions of the Green Belt techniques, concern themselves with speed and timing as their focus.

The most obvious element of structure in the system exists in the form of the Web of Knowledge. This is the evolution in attack from least serious to most serious and the relationship within and between the various techniques. For example, The first technique in each belt level deals with a **grab** as an attack, the second deals with a **push**, the third with a **punch**, the fourth with a **kick**, the fifth technique with a **hug** or a **hold**, the sixth with a **lock** or a **choke**, and the seventh with a **weapons attack**. After the first seven techniques, the web of knowledge repeats with occasional shifts of emphasis and category. This contrasts with many other ways of arranging techniques within a system and is much more logical, providing the most comprehensive coverage to the student of the art. An arrangement in which the techniques are grouped according to attack by belt level, for example, is one in which an Orange Belt might be terribly proficient at dealing with a certain type of grabbing attack while completely untrained in kicking counters. The web ensures that this will not happen.

In the 24 system of techniques found within Wu Shen Pai Kenpo, there is also a structural meaning within the 24 order. The first eight techniques comprise an orderly review of the key concepts and principles covered within earlier belt levels. The middle eight techniques in each belt serve to exhaustively explore the theme of the belt. The last eight techniques in each belt serve as either the root technique of a family group or they serve as a linkage with existing family groups. They also presage the upcoming theme by way of preparation.

Within the 24 system of technique organization, it is possible to discern an order and structure that, if followed, leads the instructor rather readily toward the development of excellence within his or her students. This is not to say that instructors within other structural arrangements of the Kenpo system cannot produce excellence. It is merely that the standardization of this more efficient structural arrangement allows for the standardization of a measure of quality control as well. Those instructors thoroughly acquainted with the themes of the belts, the arrangement and purpose of the web of knowledge, the dominant themes of the techniques, the themes of the various forms and sets, and the "whys" of the techniques, forms and sets will be able to maintain a high qualitative standard. On the other hand, those instructors without this depth of knowledge will be challenged to maintain higher qualitative standards. The modern Wu Shen Pai Kenpo system has been structured so as to eliminate guess work in matters of curriculum. There is a logical, systematic progression in which concepts, principles, theories, and definitions are explored throughout each belt level. This logical progression is the reason for the creation of the modern Wu Shen Pai Kenpo system. The member schools of the International Kenpo Karate Society that teach the Wu Shen Pai Kenpo system preserve this ordering of the techniques in order to utilize the advantages which teaching Kenpo in this systematic progression of motion offers. A familiarity with the system architecture in the form of Master Key Techniques, as well as other patterns that fall within the self defense techniques of the system, would serve to eliminate training time with the self defense techniques as well as a knowledge of Master Keys serves to eliminate training repetition in the fundamentals. There are, for example, those who might argue that the repetition of technique patterns on both sides would be necessary. It is only necessary to understand the underlying patterns of motion within the art to understand that this is unnecessary. Thrusting Salute is merely Deflecting Hammer on the opposite side. Buckling Branch is merely the opposite and reverse of Checking the Storm. There are many such patterns within the system which further serve to eliminate the need for practicing repetitious patterns. For every concept, principle, theory, definition, and movement in Wu Shen Pai Kenpo, there is an opposite and a reverse.

Chapter Four: Master Key Movements

Master Key Movements relate to the **Angle of Scaption** and the natural axis of rotation for the arms and legs. All basics, movements, techniques and Methods of execution must fall within this **Angle of Scaption**. This **Angle of Scaption** references a forty-five degree angle for both the hip and the shoulder which allow for maximum efficiency in any motion performed along this path. This angle is more efficient since it does not employ dynamic tension in the movement of the limbs. The arm, when lifted sideways, is able to execute its movement because of the expansion of the muscle under the arm and the contraction of the triceps and biceps as adductors. This tension means a reduction in speed since the arm is moving as a result of the controlled tension between these two muscle groups. This does not hold true when arm movements, or leg movements, proceed along the **Angle of Scaption**. Rather, what happens in this instance is the use of "**Gravitational Fall**" along the "groove" of the ball and socket joint which is the shoulder. Hence greater speed is enjoined to the limb since no muscle tension is required to drop the arm, only to raise or suspend it. This holds true for both the hip and the shoulder in light of the similarity which both joints have in terms of being ball and socket mechanisms. Since the basis of understanding this motion lies in the inherent biological limitations and advantages of the ball and socket joint itself, then it might be said that this principle of motion is truly universal in character. These

Master Key Movements may be categorized as either **Foot and Leg** when they involve the movement of the hips along the **Angle of Scaption** or **Hand and Arm** when they reference movement of the shoulder along the **Angle of Scaption**. **Hand and Arm** or **Foot and Leg Master Key Movements** may be further categorized as either **Right** or **Left**. When a **Foot and Leg Master Key Movement** or a **Hand and Arm Master Key Movement** are executed with either the right or the left side, the movement can be further broken down within each of these categories as being either **Clockwise** or **Counter-Clockwise**. Diagram A (below) illustrates the categorical break down of the **Master Key Movements**.

Diagram A

Counter Clockwise

Right

Clockwise

Hand and Arm Master Key Movements

Counter Clockwise

Left

Clockwise

As we come to an understanding of Master Key Movements through our grasp of the physiological and anatomical basis for the Movements, we are led to a deeper appreciation for stance, or position, within the Eight Considerations of attack and defense.   Since **Master Key Movements** have to do with **the Angle of Scaption** and the movement of the arms, or the legs, along that line, our position will determine weather we can obtain the forty-five degree angle relative to the opponent necessary to obtain the **Angle of Scaption**.   However, whether one is a practitioner of modern American Wu Shen Pai Kenpo or a tennis player, the universal character of the utilization of these paths and angles of motion within the hips and shoulders mean greater speed, power, and overall efficiency when we choose to take advantage of them to achieve **Proper Body Alignment**. Figures 38 and 39 illustrate the **Hand and Arm Master Key Movement** on the **Right Hand and Arm, Counter-Clockwise**.

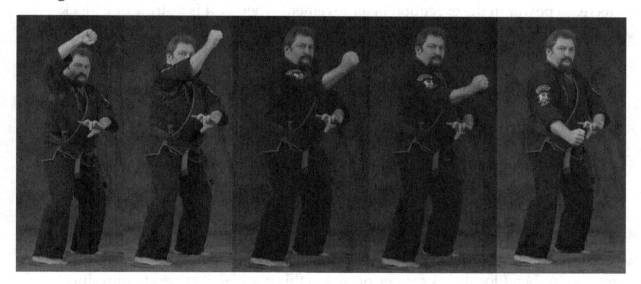

Figure 38

Figure 39

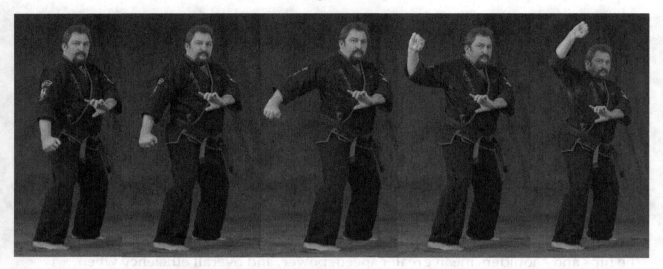

As figures 38 and 39 illustrate, all movements executed in the Wu Shen

Pai Kenpo System are executed on this path of action known as the Angle of

Scaption. Without this angle, **Improper Body Alignment** serves to significantly

decrease power in the execution of a movement whether it is a strike or a block.

It is instructive to note that the simple Yellow Belt set known as **Blocking**

Set One may be said to contain an index to the **Master Key Movements**. This set,

when performed symmetrically as it is properly performed within the Wu Shen

Pai Kenpo System, forms a basis for understanding both **Forward, Reverse**, and

Opposite forms of motion conceptually. The set is performed symmetrically;

right to left down, then reverse. This is followed by left to right down, and then

reverse. When Blocking Set is performed in this manner, it serves to introduce

the student of Wu Shen Pai Kenpo to **Master Key Movements** in the upper body,

both right and left, **Opposite** motion, **Forward** motion and **Reverse** motion. This

simple set also contains the **Master Key Positions, Master Key Methods of**

Execution, and several **Master Key Patterns**. Obviously, it is also possible to view Blocking Set One done with the lower body as illustrative of these same principles applied to the foot and leg. From salutation posture, Figures 40 and 41 illustrate the first quarter of Blocking Set One as it is practiced in the Wu Shen Pai Kenpo System. Figure 40 shows the right side of the set executed traveling downward.

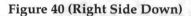

Figure 40 (Right Side Down)

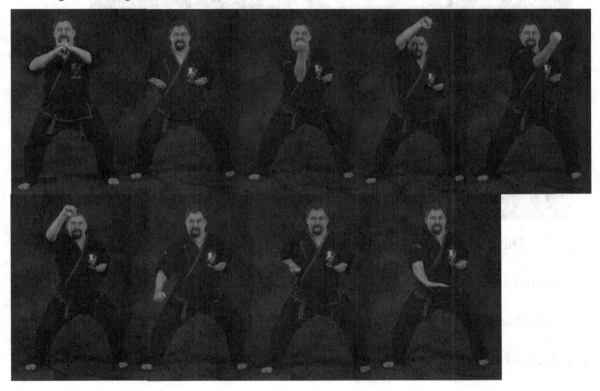

It may be readily observed from this segment of the set, that Blocking Set generally follows the contours of the **Master Key Movement** with the right side traveling counter-clockwise. The set teaches **Continuity of Motion, Proper Angles of Execution**, and **Economy of Motion** among many fundamental concepts and principles which the beginning student of Kenpo may learn. Figure

41 shows Blocking Set One, left side traveling downward which is the start of the second segment of the set.

Figure 41 (Left Side Down)

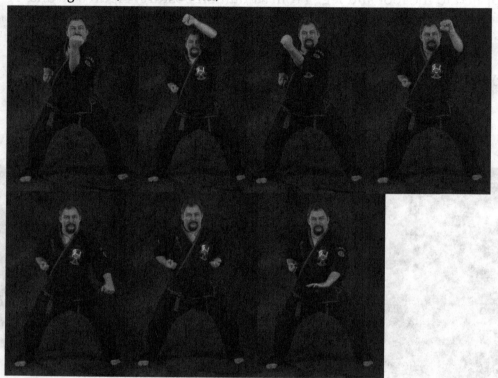

The left side traveling downward in this segment of Blocking Set One contours the lines of the **Master Key Movement** from the Left Hand and Arm, Clockwise. Figure 42 shows the right side traveling upward in the set. Other aspects of motion that the set teaches include **Master Key Positions**, or the positions our arms and hands assume prior to the execution of a **Master Key Method of Execution**. Blocking Set One also contains the **Master Key Methods of Execution Whip, Lift, Hammer, and Thrust**. For example, to reach the Upward Block in the set, it is necessary to use the **Master Key Method of Execution Lift**. The Upward Block is the **Master Key Position** for the **Master**

Key Method of Execution Hammer in this context. Lift quickly turns to **Hammer** with the Hammering Inward Block. The Inward Block is the starting point or the **Master Key Position** for the **Master Key Method of Execution Whip**. Hammer turns to Whip when we execute the Extended Outward Block segment of the set. Whip is also the **Master Key Method of Execution** for the Downward Block segment of the set. The hand on the hip becomes the **Master Key Position** for the **Master Key Method of Execution Thrust** as we execute the Push Down Block segment of the set.

Figure 42 (Right Side Traveling Upward)

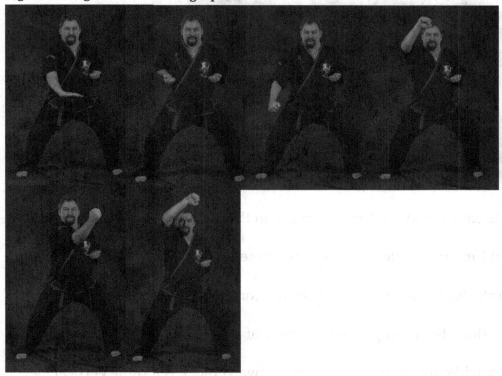

As we execute the set on the right side traveling upward, or the left side for that matter, we see the diamond as a **Master Key Pattern** which is executed both from the Downward Block going upward to the Inward Block and from the

Inward Block moving into the Upward Block.

Figure 43 (Left Side Traveling Upward)

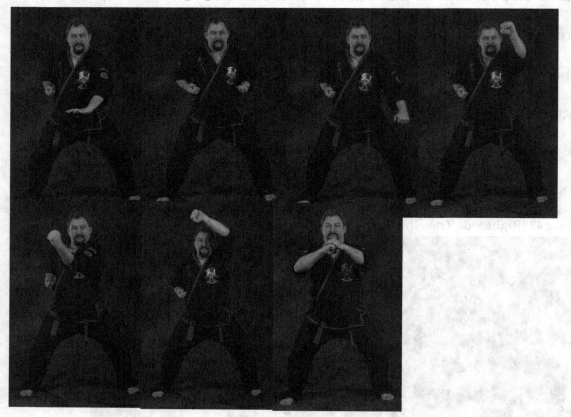

This is considered the half way mark in the execution of Blocking Set as

Wu Shen Pai Kenpo executes it. Teaching the set in this manner enables Blocking

Set to illustrate, for the student of the art, the concepts of "opposite" and

"reverse" motion. For example, the opposite of a right Inward Block is a left

Inward Block while the reverse of the right Inward Block is a right Vertical

Outward Block. These concepts are often misunderstood. The base side of the

set is right to left, that is with the right side leading and the left following the

right side in the execution of the motion and then the reverse motion is executed in the same fashion or right to left. Following the salutation posture, the opposite side of Blocking Set is then executed. The set will now be executed left to right, that is with the left side leading and the right side following the left in the execution of the motion. This segment of the set is executed moving from Left to Right, traveling down. Figure 44 illustrates the First quarter of the Left or Opposite Side of Blocking Set, traveling down.

Figure 44 (Left Side Down, Opposite Side)

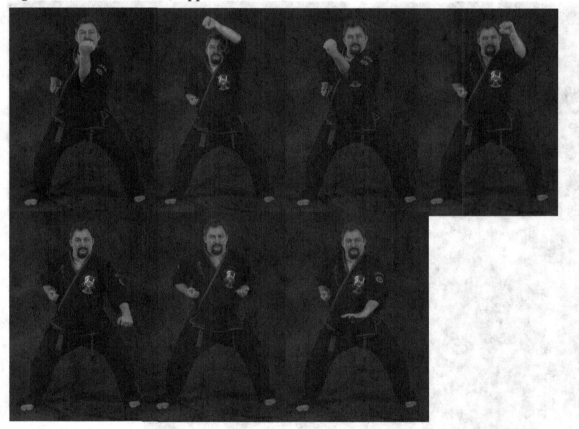

When we examine the set from the context of the **Master Key Movement,** it becomes very important to teach the concepts involved in forward and reverse motion. We come to understand, through **Master Key Forms and Sets** such as Blocking Set and through the self-defense techniques, that one element of the mastery of the art which is largely overlooked is an assessment of the Master Key Movement. The basic fundamentals which together constitute the various self-defense techniques are merely points along the path of action which is the **Master Key Movement**. Figure 45 shows Blocking Set One, Left to Right, Right Side Down which contours the Master Key Movement Right Hand and Arm, Counter-Clockwise.

Figure 45 (Right Side Down, Opposite Side)

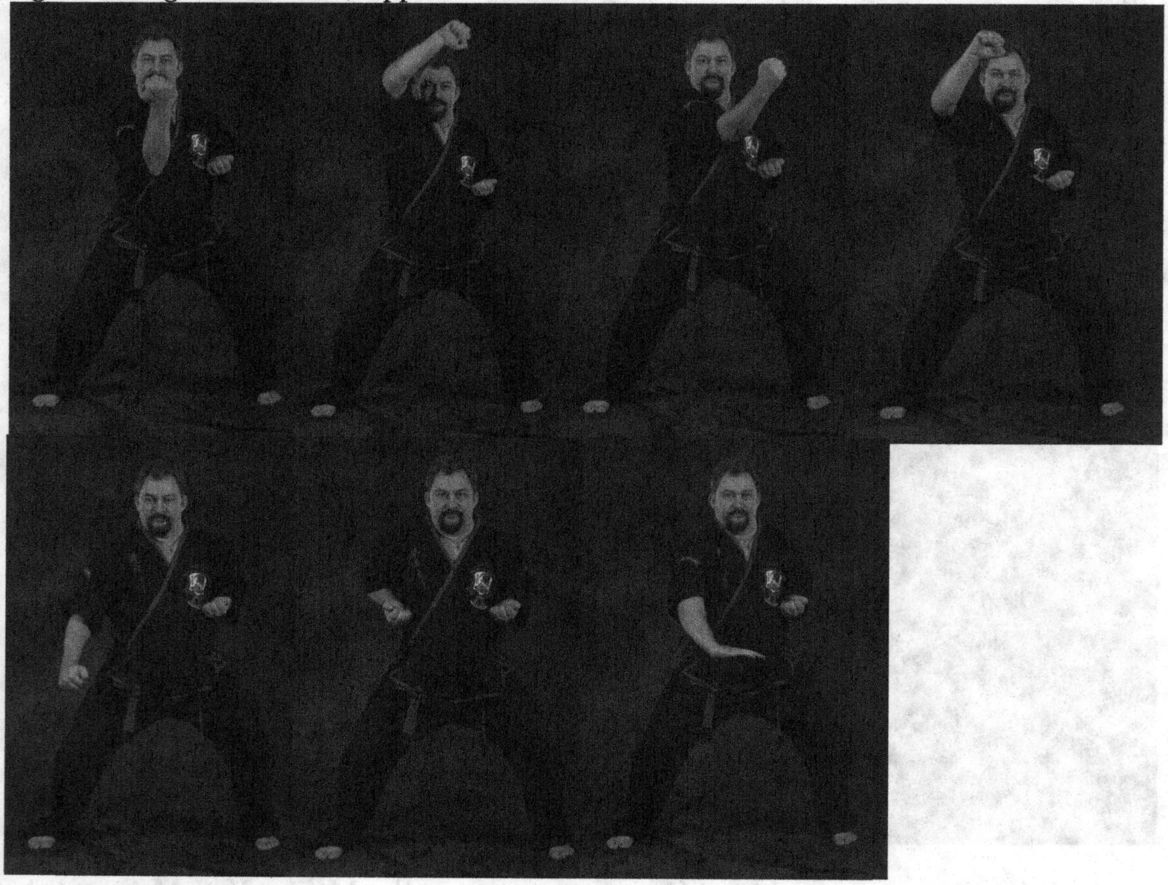

The reverse motion of the opposite side contours the **Master Key Movement** Left Hand and Arm, Clockwise. Blocking set also shows us that between each block is an Inward Block. This is true whether we examine the set traveling up or down, right or left. Figure 46 examines the Reverse motion of the set or Left Side Traveling Upward.

Figure 46 (Left Side Up, Opposite Side)

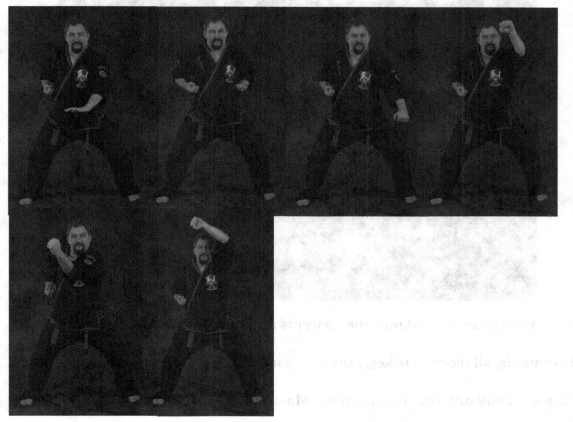

The final element of the set is the opposite side, right side traveling upward. The set will be, when performed in this manner, symmetrical. That is to say that it will be the same performed forward or reverse. When we perform this segment of the set, it contours the **Master Key Movement** Right Hand and Arm, Clockwise. Figure 47 illustrates the final segment of the **Master Key Set**, Blocking Set One.

Figure 47 (Opposite Side, Right Side Up)

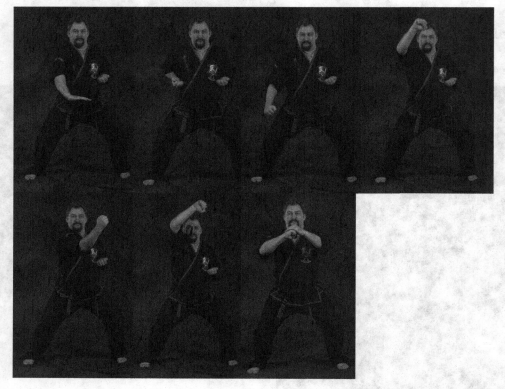

When one understands the concepts involved with **Master Key**

Movements, all blocks, strikes, punches, parries, finger techniques, and kicks

become merely differing points on the **Master Key Movement's** circular path of

action. Not only is this a highly significant concept to master for the student of

Wu Shen Pai or the martial arts in general, it is also the most significant concept

that this **Master Key Set, Blocking Set One**, communicates. Understanding and

mastering this concept means that the basic fundamentals become more useful

tools in the hands of the student. Also, fundamental concepts and principles

such as Proper Body Alignment are brought into their proper perspective.

Another interesting point of illustration within the Wu Shen Pai Kenpo

system is the entire logic surrounding the twelve Yellow Belt Techniques. These twelve techniques might be said to reference **Master Key Movements** in a number of ways. The **Master Key Movement** might be modeled from the context of the first movement in the first five Yellow Belt techniques. These techniques are Delayed Sword, Alternating Maces, Sword of Destruction, Deflecting Hammer, and Captured Twigs as taught within the Wu Shen Pai Kenpo System. Within the first hand and arm movements of these techniques is encoded the **Master Key Movement**. Illustrated in Figure 48 are the first hand and arm movements of Delayed Sword and Alternating Maces. You will observe that these two techniques, in their initial movements, represent two points on the circle of the Master Key Movement.

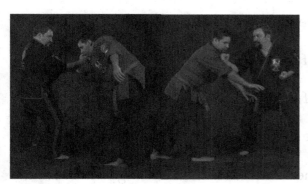

Figure 48

Comparing the techniques of the Yellow Belt based solely on the first movement, Deflecting Hammer becomes a point farther down the circle where Delayed Sword and Alternating maces precede it. Captured Twigs completes the points on the circle of the **Master Key Movement** Right Side, Counter-Clockwise. Sword of Destruction is merely another point further up, rather than down, the circle. Within the remaining seven Yellow Belt techniques is an exploration of the **Master Key Movement** from multiple perspectives. The first five techniques examine the **Master Key Movement** from a static perspective.

When we closely examine the twelve Yellow Belt techniques taught in Wu Shen Pai Kenpo we can see the **Master Key Movement** clearly defined and elaborated. There is a clear path of action that is defined in the first moves of the techniques, taken as a whole, upon which the various blocks or strikes become merely points on a circle. For example, Delayed Sword really executes the same movement pattern as Alternating Maces and Sword of Destruction, The blocks employed progressively travel around the circle. This also holds for Deflecting Hammer and Captured Twigs if we eliminate the footwork and angles employed to evade the attack and consider only the movements and position of the blocking arm. The first five technique of the Wu Shen Pai Yellow Belt curriculum entail a static examination of the Master Key Movement. Grasp of Death explores the circle and the reverse motion of the circle by coming up the circle counter clockwise and pinching the sciatica and then circling back around clockwise and executing the balance of the technique, the elbow break with the left arm. So this technique becomes an exploration of the **Master Key Movement** with the left hand and arm that is accomplished without the stopping points on the circle that characterize the first five Yellow Belt techniques. The Grasp of Death views the **Master Key Movement** from the Left Side, Clockwise from a dynamic perspective.

A dynamic examination of the Master Key Movement may be further understood through the technique Checking the Storm, once again utilizing the left hand. While Checking the Storm approaches the Master Key Movement from the dynamic perspective on the Left Side, Counter Clockwise, double factoring the block with the right arm allows us to explore the use of the Angle of Scaption, and the Master Key Movement with the right arm, Counter-Clockwise in a dynamic rather than static fashion simultaneously in this technique. Yet another dynamic exploration of the Master Key Movement is accomplished on the right side through the initial movement of the Wu Shen Pai Yellow Belt technique Mace of Aggression as illustrated in Figure 49. Another illustration of the Master Key Movement in action may be observed through the model of the Orange Belt technique Lone Kimono, as illustrated in Figure 50. In this case, the Master Key Movement is executed dynamically, Right Side, Counter Clockwise.

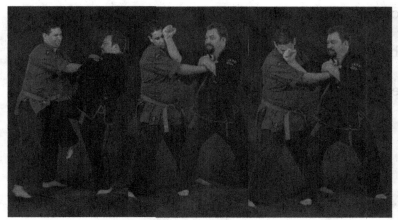

Figure 49

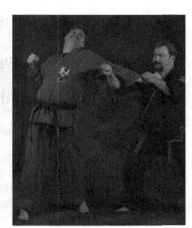

Figure 50

As you might readily observe, these techniques are merely the reverse motion of each other as they explore the Master Key Movement. Mace of

Aggression explores the Master Key Movement on right side moving counter clockwise down the circle. On the other hand, Lone Kimono explores the Master Key Movement from the right side moving clockwise up the circle.

The remaining Yellow Belt techniques in the Wu Shen Pai curriculum explore this concept as well. Attacking Mace may be readily understood as the opposite side of Delayed Sword in terms of a static examination of the Master Key Movement on the left side. Aggressive Twins repeats the emphasis of Alternating Maces with respect to this concept, only the retaliation is executed with lower case motion. Intellectual Departure starts at the down side of the circle and explores, in a dynamic fashion, the lower half of the circle upon which the **Master Key Movement** is founded. Sword and Hammer becomes a clockwise examination with the right hand of the dynamic travel up the circle and then down the circle in a path of action to conclude the technique.

In any event, the thorough understanding of the **Master Key Movement** and its exploration throughout the Kenpo Yellow Belt enables us to more thoroughly understand the roots of our motion and how it may aid us in combat.

Chapter Five: Master Key Methods of Execution

Master Key Methods of Execution refer to the manner in which a particular basic is executed in order to generate power. This can be done with **Lift, Thrust, Hammer, and Whip** or combinations of the four. Lift is the engine which drives all the other **Master Key Methods of Execution** and consequently the first which we will examine. **Lift**, as is true of all the **Master Key Methods of Execution**, can be generated with the upper body (Hand and Arm) or with the lower body (Foot and Leg). Figure 51 illustrates the end segment of the Purple Belt Wu Shen Pai technique Spiraling Twig which utilizes the **Master Key Method of Execution Lift**.

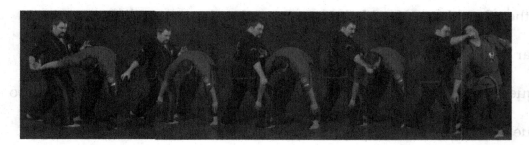

Figure 51

Lift, when executed with the foot and leg, is fairly common. For example, every time kicking is accomplished, it is done with lift. It would be impossible to effectively execute any kick without first raising the knee. This would be impossible without lift. One example of lift, executed with the foot and leg, would be the stiff leg lift kick. This kick, illustrated in Figure 52, begins from the ground and lifts straight up toward a target, typically the head or the groin, on a

given path of action.

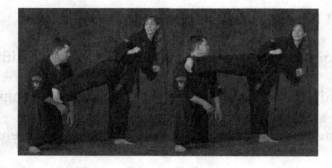

Figure 52

Whether executed with the hand and arm, or the foot and leg, the Master

Key Method of execution known as Lift is extremely important. It may be said to

be the driving force behind the other Master Key Methods of Execution. When

the Master Key Method of Execution Lift is properly understood to be the engine

behind the other Master Key Methods of Execution, important differences begin

to appear in the manner in which we execute some of our Master Key

Techniques. For example, we might look to a segment in the Wu Shen Pai Kenpo

technique Five Swords. In the segment, illustrated below in Figure 53, the right

hand is held at the Master Key Position for Lift when we initiate the execution of

our right uppercut to the Solar Plexus. This Point of Origin enhances our

striking power and differs from the more conventional approach of cocking the

hand in the Master Key Position for Thrust prior to the initiation of the same

sequence. Figure 53 illustrates the preferred position for the right hand. This

position enables us to execute Lift or graft Lift to Thrust as our Master Key

Method of Execution. Pictured is the sequence from Five Swords which demonstrates the Master Key Method of Execution Lift utilizing the hand and arm. As illustrated, following the palm heel strike to the head, the hand rests on the thigh, the Master Key Position for Lift. The body rotates and the Uppercut or Inverted Punch is directed to the solar plexus or the zyphoid process. The punch in Five Swords uses the Master Key Lift grafted to Thrust when executed in this manner.

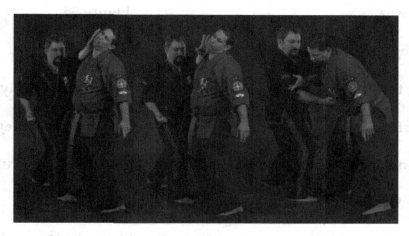

Figure 53

There is also the Master Method of Execution known as Hammer. When we execute a basic with a Hammering Method of Execution, it is very much like we are holding a hammer in hand and executing a strike. The most common method of performing an Inward Block is the Hammering Method of Execution. This is done when we perform the Wu Shen Pai forms Short Form One and Long Form One. It is also typically done when we perform the Wu Shen Pai Yellow Belt techniques "Delayed Sword" and "Alternating Maces". The Hammering Method of Execution is illustrated in Figure 54 in the initial movement of

Delayed Sword. Figure 55 illustrates a Hammering Method of Execution applied to the initial movement of Alternating Maces.

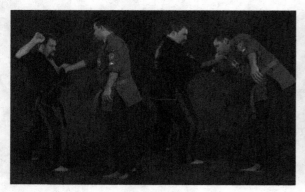

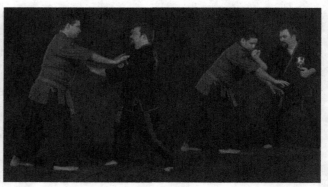

Figure 54   Figure 55

Note in the figures above the initiation of the Hammering Method of Execution utilizing the **Master Key Position for Hammering**. This is merely **Positioning for Performance** whenever we utilize this particular **Master Key Method of Execution**. Another example of the hammering method of execution is found within the **Wu Shen Pai Kenpo Yellow** belt technique Mace of Aggression. In this context, the **Hammering Master Key Method of Execution** is utilized as an Inward **Back Knuckle Rake**. This application is illustrated in Figure 56.

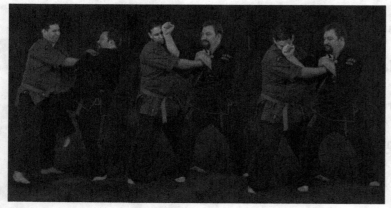

Figure 56

Another use of the Master Key Method of Execution with the Hand and Arm is when the Hammering Method of Execution is employed as an Inward Horizontal Forearm Strike against a joint. This is seen in the first movement of the Wu Shen Pai Kenpo Orange Belt technique Glancing Salute. This application

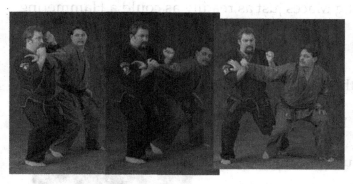

Figure 57

of the Hammering Method of Execution is shown in Figure 57 below. Not only is it possible to observe a number of different applications of a given basic within a Master Key Method of Execution, it is also possible to execute a given basic with a number of different Methods of Execution. For example, a Thrusting or a Hammering Method of Execution can be employed when performing an Inward Block. We can readily see this application of the Inward Block in the Wu Shen Pai Purple Belt technique Darting Mace. Figure 58 shows the Thrusting Master Key Method of Execution in the application of the Inward Block in the initial moves of that technique.

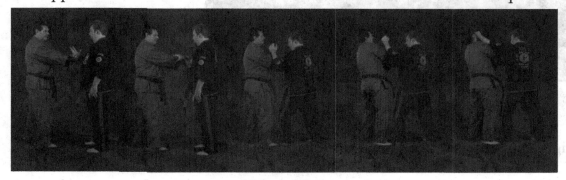

Figure 58

This is a principle that is obviously applicable to a wide range of techniques. For example, we could employ a Hammering or a Thrusting Master Key Method of Execution in the initial movement of the Wu Shen Pai Yellow Belt technique Delayed Sword. A Thrusting Method of Execution may be utilized in the initial movement of Alternating Maces just as readily as could a Hammering Method of Execution.

Whip is the final and fourth Master Key Method of Execution. Whip may be observed in a multitude of self-defense techniques in American Wu Shen Pai Kenpo. Figure 59, at right, illustrates the use of the Master Key Method of Execution known as Whip in the final movement of the Wu Shen Pai Kenpo Orange Belt technique, Lone Kimono. Also, the return, which is a major

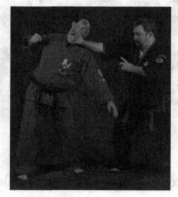

Figure 59

characteristic of whip is illustrated in the Wu Shen Pai Kenpo Yellow Belt

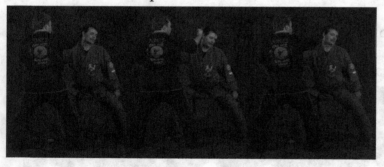

technique Checking the Storm. This may be readily observed in the sequence of Figure 60. Note that the elbow in

Figure 60

Figure 60 is cocked following the execution of the basic. This is an exaggeration of the movement, done only in the embryonic stages of development. Although one illustration of the principle Whip as a **Master Key Method of Execution**

112

utilizes an outward sword hand, and the other uses a back knuckle, both are examples of the **Master Key Method of Execution** known as **Whip**. The natural weapon used in the **Method of Execution** is of no importance and is reflective of the fit of the target to the weapon and other factors. What is significant is the actual **Master Key Method of Execution**. Understanding **Master Key Methods of Execution** enable us to use whatever we wish to use as a natural weapon to great effectiveness.

Grafting

In addition to selecting a single Master Key Method of Execution in pairing to a given basic, we might also choose to employ multiple Master Key Methods of Execution within the application of a given basic. This is known as grafting together differing Master Key Methods of Execution. We might employ these varying Methods of Execution within a given basic for a number of reasons.

When we combine the four Master Key Methods of Execution in any order, we are said to be Grafting differing Methods of Execution. It is grafting the differing methods of execution that constitutes the basis of the art and certainly the basis for mastery of the hard aspects of Exterior Power in the art of Wu Shen Pai Kenpo. It may not be a stretch to say that this concept is the basis for the mastery of all martial arts systems. We might employ differing methods of execution within the same motion of the same technique. For example, we might examine the Master Key Technique Five Swords taught in Wu Shen Pai Kenpo at the Orange Belt level. A practitioner of American Wu Shen Pai Kenpo might employ Hammer or Thrust in the initial right Inward Block movement. Given greater understanding with respect to the motion of the system, the same sequence might be executed with Hammer to Thrust as the Master Key Method of Execution. Another alternative for the execution of that same movement would be to initiate the Inward Block with the Master Key Method of Execution Lift to Hammer to Thrust. To enhance hitting power, the angular line of attack with the Outward Handsword might be rounded off to graft Whip as a suffix to the already utilized Lift to Hammer to Thrust. The reason for selection might be something as simple as personal preference or a tailored response in which the individual Kenpoist might execute the motion more effectively. It might also arise from a desire to achieve a particular effect, or even strike a particular pressure point in executing a block or strike.

The utilization of differing methods of execution within a given basic is a matter of personal choice and a function of tailoring the art to the individual. For example, some individuals derive greater power from the execution of a Whip, while others might derive greater functionality from Thrust. Consequently, grafting the two Master Keys together might be advantageous if, individually, we could obtain the advantages offered by two or more Master Key Methods of Execution within a given basic.

Accurately striking a given target more efficiently would be a strong rationale for the utilization of varying **Master Key Methods of Execution** within a given sequence. Grafting and selection of **Master Key Methods of Execution** that are appropriate to the action which needs to be performed, are aided through an understanding of the **Master Key Positions**. In other words, grafting and selection of the appropriate **Master Key Methods of Execution** are a function of the position of the hand and arm at the initiation of the action. As we come to learn, **Position** is vital. It is one of the **Eight Considerations for Attack and Defense** which we must consider in order to arrive at an accurate assessment of our self-defense scenario. There are four **Master Key Positions**. All four of these positions are illustrated in their ideal phase. Since the use of one or another of the Master Key Methods of Execution has to do with the position which one finds oneself in at the initiation of the defensive action, the analysis of these initial positions becomes important. These positions actually determine the Method of Execution of our next movement. Understanding Master Key Positions enables us to better understand where we go next in the sequences that we will employ. Greater efficiency in our motion might be realized if, given an understanding of these positions, we consciously move to a **Master Key Position** in the hope of utilizing the corresponding **Master Key Method of Execution** for the advantages it offers. Conscious efforts at intelligently utilizing new **Points of Origin** to take full advantage of Master Key Positions are known as **Positioning for Performance**. There are **four Master Key**

Positions that enable us to **Position for Performance**. These Master Key

Positions are linked to the four **Master Key Methods of Execution** already

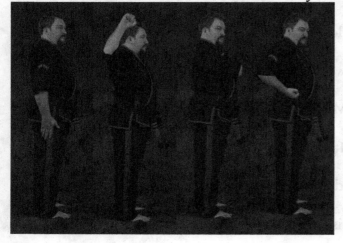

described. From left to right,

they are the Master Key Positions

for the **Master Key Methods of**

Execution Lift, Hammer, Whip,

and Thrust. These four hand

and arm **Master Key Positions**

Figure 61

are illustrated below in Figure

61. Although not illustrated, there are analogous **Master Key Positions** with the

foot and leg which lead us to the execution of a **Whipping, Thrusting, or**

Hammering Method of Execution in kicking. **Lift** is an axiomatic Master Key in

the execution of kicks. The **Master Key Position for Lift** with the foot and leg is,

therefore, axiomatic also.

Mastery of the art lies in the grafting of these differing Master Key

Methods of Execution together in order to reap the advantages that they might

offer from time to time within a given sequence. The secret to continuity of

motion and relaxation lies in the ability to graft these differing Master Key

Methods of Execution together in a smooth sequential flow. Without relaxation,

this would be all but impossible. Conversely, grafting the differing Master Key

Methods of Execution enables us to develop both the relaxation necessary to

greater speed and power, and the continuity that allows us to be flexible in our treatment of movement and motion. The importance of Master Keys may be understood more readily when we acknowledge that what we search for in the martial arts, but particularly in Wu Shen Pai Kenpo, are the overarching laws which will define for us the precise expectations for our motion and its effects. In other words, we want to be able to predict that using this or that movement will result in this or that effect. We wish to obtain for ourselves the most efficient and hence most effective solution to our self defense dilemma.

Chapter Six: Grafting Together Master Key Methods of Execution

What is Grafting?

Grafting in the medical world is taking tissue from one place and surgically affixing it to another. In motion, essentially the same process is followed. When grafting motion, one type of motion is "affixed" or attached to another type or form of motion. This gives our motion a level of variability that is virtually unlimited. Grafting together differing **Master Key Methods of Execution** are but one form of grafting together motion and it is the most profound. In the normal state of affairs a single **Master Key Method of Execution** is paired, in an embryonic state, to a single given basic. As we come to understand the subtlety and sophistication of motion, we come to realize that we might also choose to employ multiple **Master Key Methods of Execution** within the application of a given basic. This is known as **grafting** together differing **Master Key Methods of Execution**. It is probably the most essential skill to master in order to achieve mastery of **Exterior Power** in Wu Shen Pai Kenpo. It may not be a stretch to say that this concept is the basis for the mastery of all martial arts systems. As previously noted, there are a number of reasons for doing so. Fitting the **Master Key Method of Execution** to achieve greater efficiency might be one reason. It might also be appropriate to select a particular graft in order to maximize the tailoring of the movement to the practitioner. It might also arise from a desire to achieve a particular effect, or even strike a particular pressure point in executing a block or strike. The utilization of differing methods of execution within a given basic is a matter of personal choice and a function of tailoring the art to the individual.

Hand and Arm Grafts of the Master Key Methods of Execution

There are a number of ways of grafting differing Master Key Methods of Execution together in a single sequence. First, we may use the **hand and arm** to graft differing **Master Key Methods of Execution**. With the hand and arm, we may graft **Lift to Thrust, Lift to Hammer, and Lift to Whip**. We may also graft **Hammer to Lift, Hammer to Thrust, and Hammer to Whip**. We could **graft Thrust to Lift, Thrust to Hammer, and Thrust to Whip**. Finally, we could graft **Whip to Hammer, Whip to Lift, and Whip to Thrust**.

Grafting Lift to Thrust with the hand and arm is observed in the Wu Shen Pai Purple Belt self defense technique Thundering Hammers. These are illustrated below in Figure 62. In the first two segments of the illustration, the

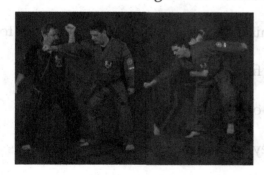

two movements of the technique itself are shown. The arm positions illustrating the **Master Key Position for Lift** and the end position where **Thrust** has clearly occurred are shown.

Figure 62

Another technique which illustrates a graft between the Master Key Methods of Execution Lift to Thrust is the Wu Shen Pai Orange belt technique common to many systems of Kenpo known as Dance of Death. Figure 63 shows

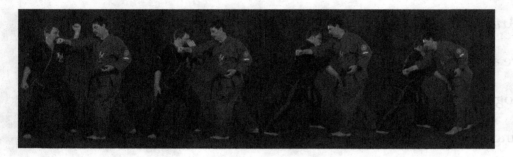

Figure 63

from left to right the point of origin indicative of Lift being next utilized as a Master Key Method of Execution, moving to a Thrusting Master Key Method of Execution, and finally the actual execution of Thrust. Lift to Hammer might be observed in the initial moves of the Yellow Belt technique Alternating Maces. It is also found, more obviously, in the first few movements of the Wu Shen Pai Kenpo Orange Belt technique Lone Kimono, as shown in Figure 64. It is also possible to execute a three-way graft with this technique sequence grafting Lift to Hammer to Whip as is illustrated in the last frames of the same figure. The subtlety of grafting these differing Methods of Execution is readily observed in the above sequence. Grafting two Master Key Methods of Execution together, as we are illustrating in this chapter, is merely one dimension of the concept. We might choose to graft two, three, or even four, Master Key Methods of Execution together in a single sequence of motion.

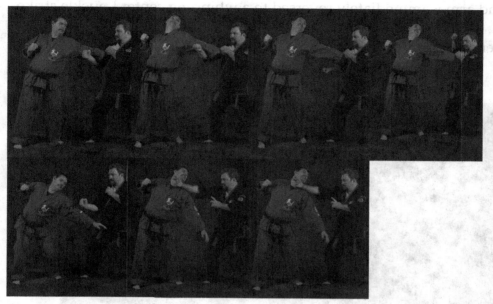

Figure 64

This notion of grafting more than two Master Key Methods of Execution as illustrated in Figure 64 above through the model of Lone Kimono is but one illustration of the concept. Grafting of differing Master Key Methods of Execution is so crucial to the mastery of the art since it may be accomplished in a myriad of ways and does not merely occur one dimensionally. Such grafting may occur within each sequence of a given technique enhancing the effectiveness of the motion by using the grafting to enhance the striking power of the sequence. A graft may increase the speed of the strike, block, or both thus enhancing its power.

The graft between Lift to Whip is observed through the Green Belt technique Obscure Claws. As we view Figure 65 from left to right the opponent is struck from behind with a right looping overhead punch, the motion of the right hand and arm is immediately reversed to a whipping center knuckle strike to the opponent's sternum.

Figure 65

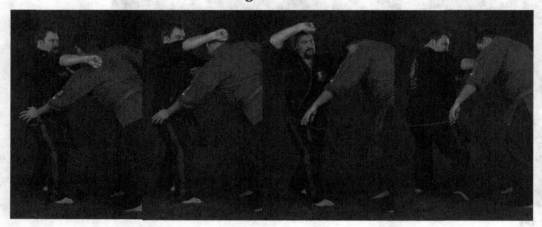

We may also graft Hammer to Lift as evidenced in the extension to the Wu Shen Pai Orange Belt Technique Five Swords. Illustrated below in Figure 66 are the Master Key Methods of Execution Hammer to Lift grafted in the model of the Orange Belt technique Five Swords. Notice the right hand as it passes through the neck as the target and rebounds back to strike the throat grafting the Master Key Method of execution Hammer to Lift as the Outward Handsword to the throat is administered.

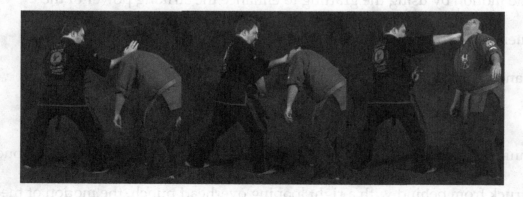

Figure 66

The graft between the Master Methods of Execution Hammer to Thrust is best observed in the Wu Shen Pai Purple Belt technique Darting Mace. In this case, the effectiveness of the graft is enhanced by its use of a pressure point to affect the opponent. Figure 67, below, shows this graft.

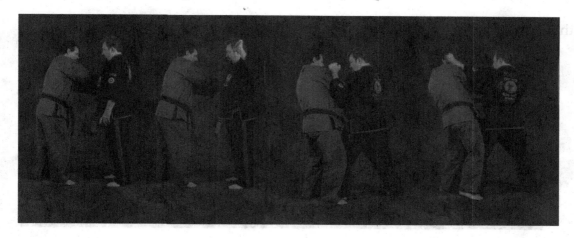

Figure 67

Hammer to Whip is observed in the initial movements of Delayed Sword as we execute a Hammering Inward block followed immediately by the Outward Handsword executed with the utilization of the Master Key Method of Execution Whip. Figure 68 illustrates this graft in its more embryonic state.

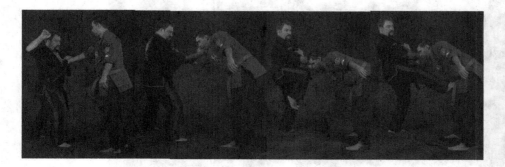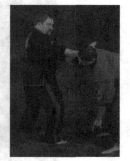

Figure 68

We could observe how to execute the graft of the Master Key Methods of Execution Thrust to Lift through a careful examination of the Wu Shen Pai 1st Degree Brown Belt Technique Thrusting Salute. This is illustrated in Figure 69 below. This extension is but one of many that serve as grafting models for our further education in, or "extension" of, the concepts and principles of motion.

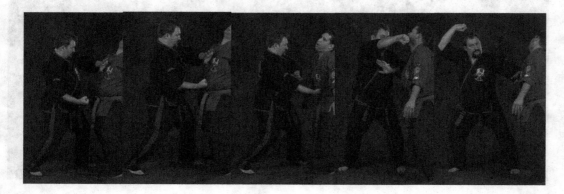

Figure 69

Thrust to Hammer is a concept clearly illustrated in the extension to the Wu Shen Pai Kenpo technique Five Swords as shown in Figure 70. After the Right Uppercut, the right hand rebounds and circles, grafting to a Hammering Inward Hand Sword.

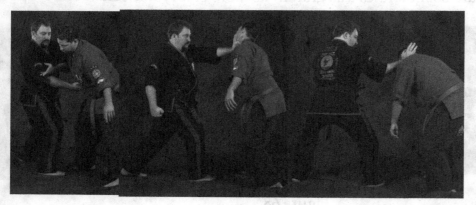

Figure 70

Thrust to Whip as a concept is also demonstrated in the technique Five Swords. Instead of focusing on the right hand, focus on the left. As illustrated in Figure 71, following the left Thrusting Palm Heel, the left hand rebounds from the right bicep and grafts into a Whipping Outward Hand Sword to the neck/mastoid area.

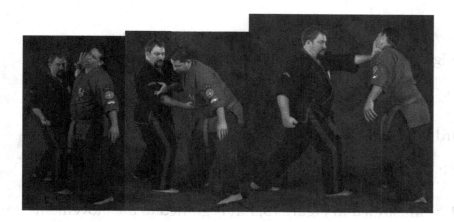

Figure 71

Finally, when consider Hand and Arm grafts of the Master Key Methods of Execution, we could observe the graft of Whip to Hammer. Figure 72 shows this particular graft modeled for us in the Wu Shen Pai Blue Belt technique Shield and Mace. The first portion of the technique, shown here in the first segments of Figure 72, illustrates a right Vertical Outward Parry using the Master Key Method of Execution Whip. Immediately following this action, the right hand reverses, as shown, and strikes the opponent's right kidney. This employs the Master Key Method of Execution Hammer.

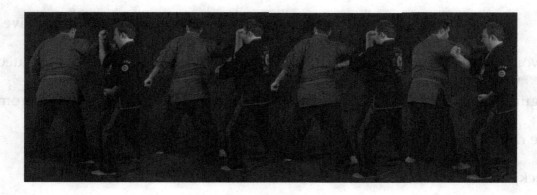

Figure 72

Whip to Lift might be best understood through the model of Five Swords. After blocking with the a right Inward Block and a left Outward Handsword check, a right Outward Whipping Handsword to the appropriate pressure points is initiated. As the right hand flows through the target and following the Left Thrusting Palm Heel, as illustrated in Figure 73, Lift is grafted to the movement to initiate the right Uppercut.

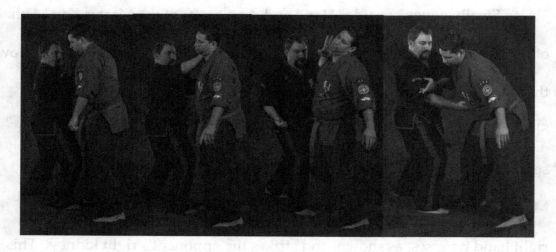

Figure 73

Whip to Thrust might be understood through an assessment of the motion ending Checking The Storm, a Wu Shen Pai Yellow Belt technique. The back knuckle, as illustrated in Figure 74, is retracted and thrust is initiated by the insertion of an

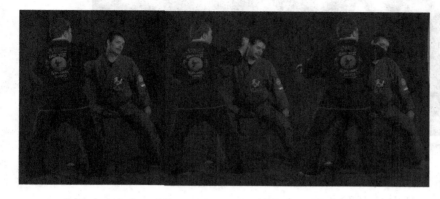

Figure 74

Inward Horizontal

Elbow striking to the

head or jaw.

Grafting the differing Master Key Methods of Execution occurs throughout the Wu Shen Pai Kenpo system in a multitude of settings. It may be initiated because the action requires it, or grafting of this sort may occur as a conscious choice in an effort to tailor the motion to the individual or to gain the advantages offered by a particular Master Key Method of Execution.

Foot and Leg Grafts of the Master Key Methods of Execution

Another method of grafting the differing Master Key Methods of Execution together involves those motions utilizing the foot and leg. With the foot and leg, we could graft **Lift to Whip, Lift to Thrust, and Lift to Hammer**. **Lift** occurs when we raise the knee to the Master Key for Kicking. From this point, we could execute a Front Snap Ball Kick, or a Roundhouse Snap Kick, effectively grafting **Lift to Whip**. This is shown applied in the Wu Shen Pai Yellow Belt Technique Attacking Mace in Figure 75.

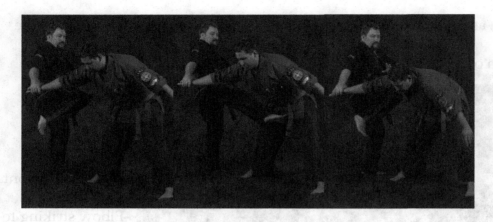

Figure 75

The Wu Shen Pai Purple Belt Self-Defense technique Spiraling Twigs is the model for yet another graft of Lift to Thrust. From the Master Key For Kicking, which we use as a reference point we may execute a Front Thrust Kick, and consequently graft **Lift to Thrust.**

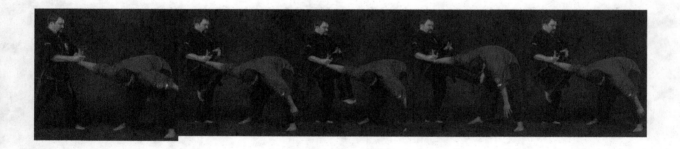

Figure 76

Lift to Hammer is seen to occur in the 3rd Degree Black Belt extension to the Wu Shen Pai Green Belt technique Intercepting the Ram. This is illustrated below in Figure 77. **Whip to Lift** is illustrated in the initial moves of this technique where a scoop kick is executed to the opponent's jaw, while **Lift to Hammer** is clearly shown in the final kick which is a Jump Inside Crescent Kick.

128

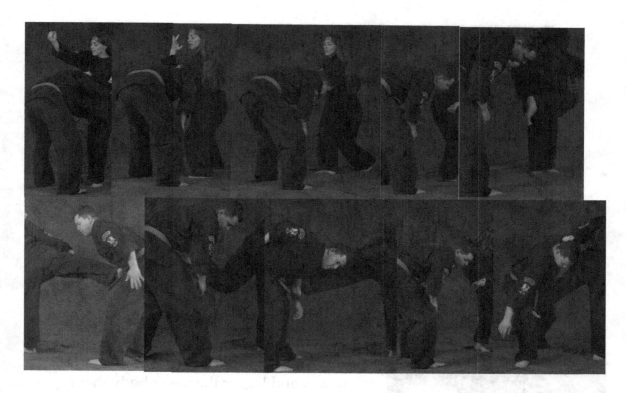

Figure 77

We could also graft, with Lift assumed, **Whip to Thrust**. Figure 78 shows

this graft in the Wu Shen Pai 3rd Degree Black Belt technique Leap From Danger.

Shown are the final movements of the extension to this Green Belt technique

where a low Heel Hook Kick (Whip) to the back of the opponent's knee is grafted

within the same movement to a Roundhouse Thrust Kick to the Chest (Thrust).

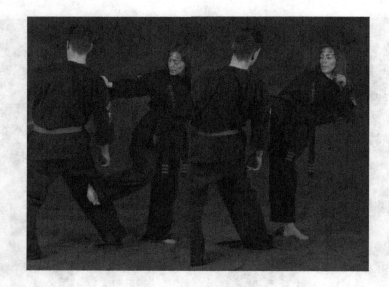

Figure 78

Whip to Hammer is another possible graft of the foot and leg, or the lower body that is illustrated in Figure 79 at left. Shown is the Right Knife Edge Kick followed by the Right Inward Sweep in the Wu Shen Pai 3rd Degree Brown Belt Technique Prance of the Tiger. The difference

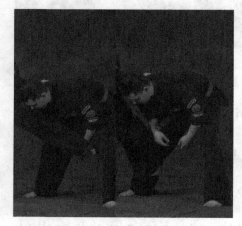

Figure 79

between this application of the two movements is what defines the Master Key Methods of Execution. As it is executed in Wu Shen Pai, instead of a Thrusting Sweep Kick as in the technique Unfolding the Dark, a Hammering Master Key Method of Execution is used instead effecting a more efficient sweep as a result. This, in part, is because the order of the execution is reversed in this instance.

Another possible graft of differing Master Key Methods of Execution with the foot and leg is **Hammer to Thrust**. This graft occurs in the Wu Shen Pai 3rd

Degree Black Belt technique Intercepting the Ram at the very end. This graft is

illustrated in Figure 80. The entire sequence is illustrated in Figure 77.

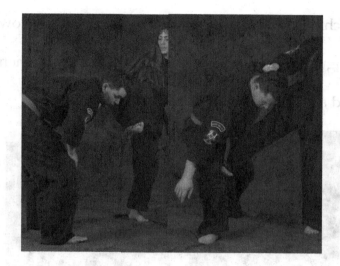

Figure 80

Hammer to Whip where Lift is assumed to occur is yet another graft of

the foot and leg. This is shown in Figure 81. This occurs when the right leg

executes a Right Outside Full Moon Kick and rebounds from the ground and

directly into a graft of the Master Key Method of Execution Thrust in the

execution of a Roundhouse Thrust Kick.

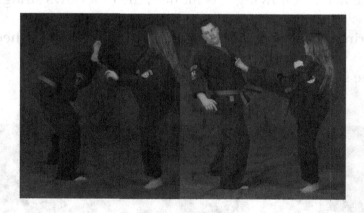

Figure 81

Thrust to Lift is found grafted in a multitude of techniques. One place where such a graft is located is the 3rd Degree Brown Belt technique Courting the Tiger in the last movement of the technique. This is illustrated in the abstract below in Figure 82. The last frame of Figure 82 shows the application of the graft when used in Courting the Tiger and a myriad of other Brown Belt techniques.

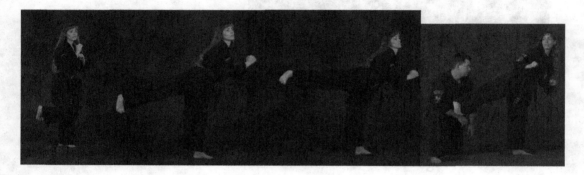

Figure 82

Thrust to Hammer is show in Figure 83. Shown Illustrated is a portion of the Wu Shen Pai Kenpo 2nd Degree Black Belt extension to the technique Circling the Horizon. From the initial frame the Master Key Thrust is used to strike the opponent's kidney with the heel. Following this motion, the foot flows straight into a graft of the Hammering Master Key Method of Execution where the heel strikes straight down to the sternum.

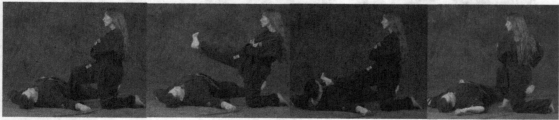

Figure 83

Thrust to Whip is illustrated by a sequence from the 3rd Degree Brown Belt technique Unfolding the Dark. After the actual takedown, a Right Thrusting Sweep Kick clears the opponent's left leg and prevents the opponent from getting up. Immediately following that, the Right Side Knife Edge Kick is directed to the opponent's throat. This sequence is shown in Figure 84, below.

Figure 84

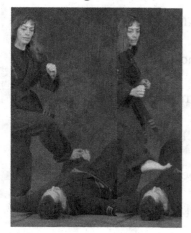

The grafting of **Master Key Methods of Execution** becomes the basis for proficiency in both striking and kicking and consequently the fundamental basis for the mastery of hard or striking portion of the art. One of the more noticeable benefits of practicing the Extensions to the base techniques in the Kenpo system is that these grafting concepts are executed for the lower body primarily within the context of those extensions. The extensions to the base techniques truly become, in Wu Shen Pai Kenpo, extensions of the concepts and principles previously studied in the base. They merely repeat the various belt themes with the lower body involved, thus completing the cycle of learning. Extensions to the base techniques, in this context, become a valuable addition to the overall understanding of body mechanics and motion inherent in the modern Wu Shen Pai system of Kenpo.

Chapter Seven: Master Key Forms and Sets

Master Key Forms

Forms in the Wu Shen Pai Kenpo system are created with the purpose of aiding the student in understanding the various concepts and principles of the art. They exist for no other reason than to model these concepts and principles of motion to aid the student in achieving mastery of them. **Master Key Forms** are forms that form the core of instruction in the concepts and principles of Wu Shen Pai Kenpo. Short Form One is one such Master Key Form. Long Form One and Long Form Two are also Master Key Forms. Long Form Four is yet another.

There are patterns in the forms that enable us to better understand their purpose as well. Short Form One, Long Form One, Short Form Two, and Long Form Two are **Dictionary Forms**. They serve to define motion and movement. They pinpoint proper form to achieve such fundamental concepts as **Proper Body Alignment**. Short Form Three, Long Form Three, are Long Form Four are **Encyclopedic Forms**. These forms place the learned concepts explored in the **Dictionary Forms** into a context, just as Encyclopedias place knowledge into context. Finally, there are **Specialized Forms**. Long Form Five and Six fall into this category which is a subcategory of **Encyclopedic Forms**. Long Form Five is a **Specialized Form** teaching strike down techniques, while Long Form Six is a **Specialized Form** teaching empty hand defenses against weapons attacks. Long

Form Seven and Long Form Eight in the Kenpo system fall into another category appropriately entitled **Weapons Forms.** Understanding this underlying structure enables us to understand what the system as a whole is trying to communicate through its forms. Wu Shen Pai also teaches traditional Chinese hand sets. Of these, Short Form of the Tiger, Movements of the Tiger, and Twist of the Tiger are considered to be Master Key Forms. They fall into the Dictionary category since they teach elements of motion definition.

Master Key Sets

Training Sets are created based upon their ability to assist the student in understanding some quality or characteristic which they should wish to obtain or upon basics which require further refinement and elaboration. These categorizations are termed **Fundamental Sets, Qualitative Sets, and Weapons Sets.** Those sets that are rooted in the basic fundamentals and their elaboration are **Fundamental Sets.** They typically isolate some aspect of training fundamental basics which may challenge the student or be of crucial importance to building further skill. For example, if the student wishes to work and train his or her stances, there is Stance Set One and Stance Set Two. If a student wishes to train and refine their blocking skills, there is Blocking Set One or Blocking Set Two. If the student wishes to refine their punching and striking skills, then there is Striking Set One and Striking Set Two. If the student wishes to further their understanding of finger techniques, then there is Finger Set One and Finger Set

Two. If the student wishes to learn more about and deepen their understanding of kicking, then there is Kicking Set One and Kicking Set Two. Parries and Foot Maneuvers are inclusive in all of the sets and thus need no further elaboration.

Qualitative Sets are so named because they serve to build a quality or characteristic which may challenge the student or which the student may build up further through additional training. For example, Coordination Set One and Coordination Set Two, while rooted in the basic fundamentals, serve to further fine tune a student's eye-hand and eye-foot coordination in a variety of ways. To further the timing skills of our students, Wu Shen Pai Kenpo teaches Timing Set One.

Weapons Sets are those sets that serve to highlight skills in a particular weapon. There is, for example, Knife Set One which teaches knife handling skills and dexterity drills for the knife preparatory to learning the more subtle motion of Long Form Eight. There is Club Set One which introduces the student to skills involved in handling the double sticks. There is also Staff Set One that also teaches fundamental staff handling skills in the context of circular motion. Wu Shen Pai Kenpo also teaches a myriad of weapons for the purpose of further refinement of body mechanics and skill sets. Tsa Kwon, for example, serves to teach pole staff handling skills not otherwise taught. The teaching of weapon sets serve another end in Wu Shen Pai. They serve to condition and strengthen the body. Chinese Broadsword sets such as Fumi Darn Dao and Plum Blossom

Darn Dao serve to build up and strengthen the wrist. Sets with the Kwan Dao serve to build upper body strength and cardiovascular conditioning.

Master Key Sets include Blocking Set One, Kicking Set One, Coordination Set One, Stance Set One, Finger Set One, Striking Set One, and Timing Set One. The Master Key Set illustrated here is Striking Set One. This set was selected since it is a Master Key Set and because of its importance in virtually every arena of training. Striking Set is utilized in training sparring traps and drills. It is used to emphasize paths and lines of motion, upper and lower case motion, and it serves to illustrate an unusual but very significant grafting of **Master Key Methods of Execution**. Striking Set One models the grafting of the Master Key Method of Execution **Thrust to** the Master Key Methods of Execution **Lift, Hammer, and Whip**. The core sequence teaches a Straight Thrust Punch (Thrust) grafted to a Horizontal Back Knuckle (Whip), then an Inverted Hammer Fist (Whip), an Inverted Vertical Punch (Lift), and finally an Inward Hammerfist (Hammer).

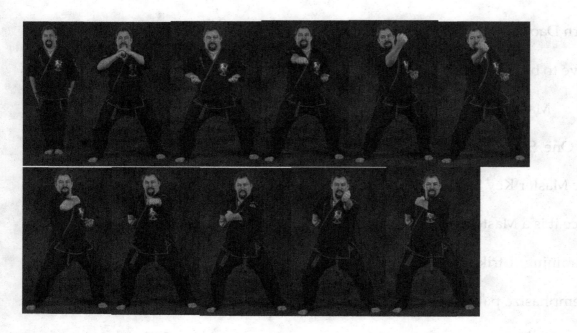

Figure 85

Figure 85 depicts the first segment of **Striking Set One,** Strikes to the

Front. Specifically, Figure 85 shows the graft of Thrust to Whip. This particular

segment also models the re-orbit from the horizontal (or z) axis of the body to the

diagonal angles of execution. An analysis of this portion of the set also entails an

understanding of **paths** versus **lines** of motion.

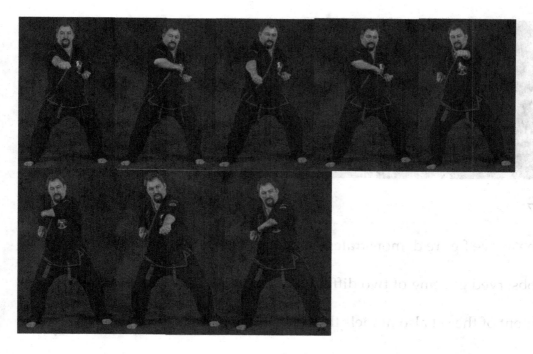

Figure 86

  The graft from **Thrust to Whip** is explored from a different angle of execution in Figure 86. This completes an X pattern of motion overlaid on a horizontal axis of motion, if we view the pattern three dimensionally. This motion teaches the use of a horizontal line of motion, possibly countered, and converted to a diagonal path of action which deceptively arrives at the target. This interpretation of the motion is what makes the set useful as a sparring drill. All that this entails is moving from the horse stance to the Neutral Bow in its execution.

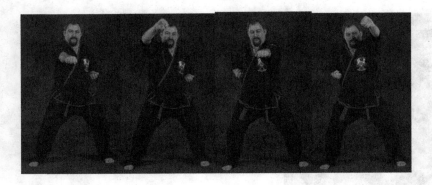

Figure 87

The above figure demonstrates the graft between **Thrust and Lift**. This is

a rarely observed grafting of two differing **Master Key Methods of Execution**.

This segment of the set also models the **Heart Shaped Pattern**, a **Master Key**

Pattern that is executed in the **Reverse Motion** or bottom to top.

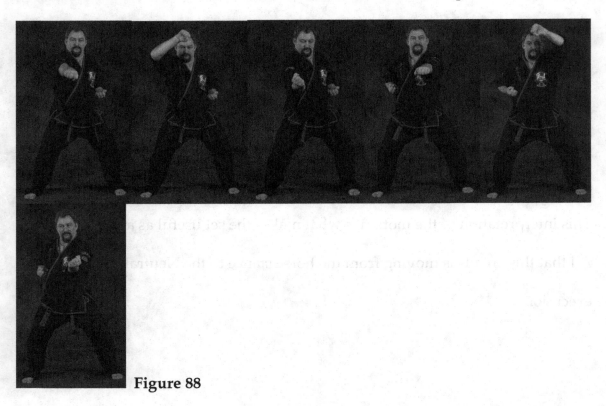

Figure 88

The previous sequence, in Figure 88, illustrates the graft between Thrust

and Hammer. This sequence also explores the **Heart Shaped Pattern** this time from **Forward Motion** or top to bottom. The next segment is the same sequence, with the exception that the punch is a vertical punch and not a straight thrust punch, executed to the sides, first to the right and then to the left.

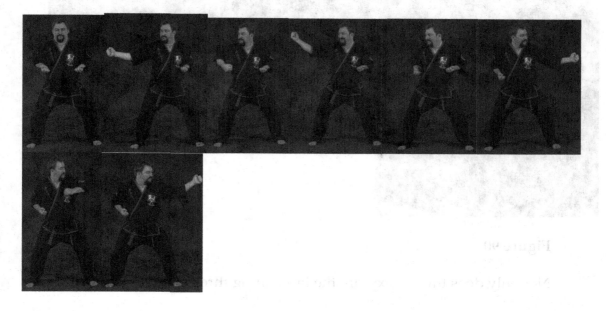

Figure 89

Strikes done to the side with this segment of Striking Set One tend to explore three-dimensional motion and the **Heart Shaped Pattern** from the horizontal plane of action as is the case with the Straight Punch to Horizontal Back Knuckle done to the front. This is an exploration of the **Half Heart Shape** from both **Forward Motion** and **Reverse Motion**. This theme of the **Heart Shaped Pattern** performed to 3 and 9 o'clock is repeated in the lower case completing the pattern as shown in Figure 90. If we view Striking Set One in a three dimensional matrix, it is interesting to observe the Master Key Patterns which emerge.

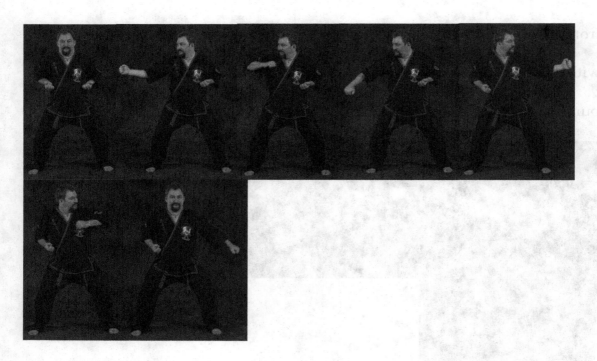

Figure 90

Not only does this set explore the fascinating three-dimensional contours

of the universal pattern, it also examines the angle of scaption as it may be

effectively utilized from a number of perspectives. Figure 91, below, shows the

elaboration of Thrust to Lift as we further explore the motion patterns of the set.

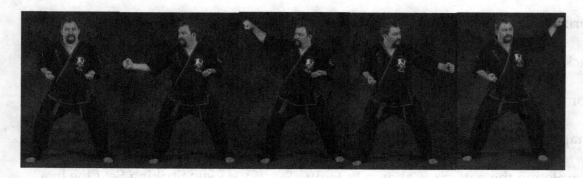

Figure 91

Figure 92 illustrates the strikes to the side grafting the Master Key

Methods of Execution Thrust to Hammer.

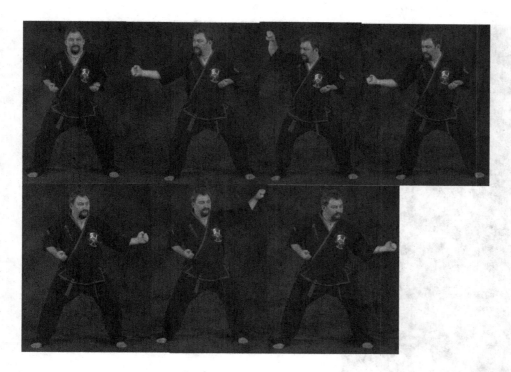

Figure 92

Once strikes to the side are completed, the next segment of the set involves

double strikes to the front and to the side. This segment of the set defines the

circle on a vertical plane of action. It also fully the explores the **Heart Shape**

Pattern, as the **Half Heart Shape** had been previously examined. Both of these

are **Master Key Patterns** of motion. These strikes also serve to teach continuity of

motion, flow, and relaxation. **Economy of Motion** is, of course, another concept

thoroughly explored in this set. Figure 93 shows double strikes to the front and

side.

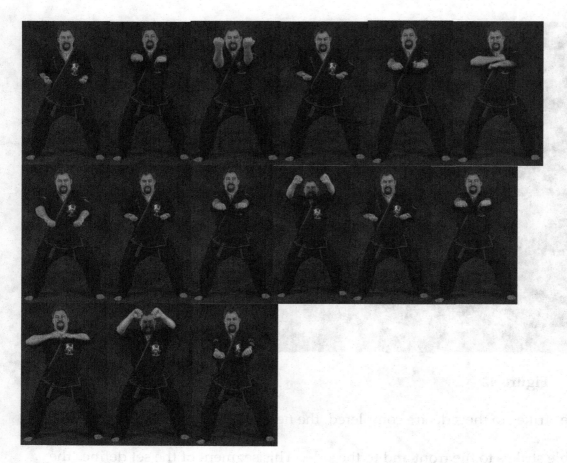

Figure 93

The next sequence of the set, shown in Figure 94, are the strikes executed

to the side right and left simultaneously. This portion of the form results in yet

another examination of the motion of the set from a three dimensional

perspective. Once again the **Heart Shape Pattern** is executed in a patch of action,

in this case horizontally to the sides. The universal pattern is viewed in this set

as a three dimensional object with the practitioner standing in the middle of the

pattern. Paths of action serve to create the patterns which are **Master Key**

Patterns of motion.

144

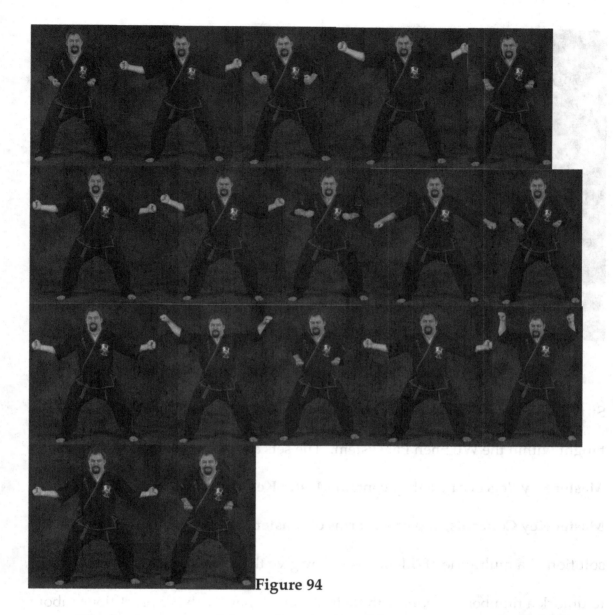

Figure 94

The final segment of the set is a reprise of the sets major strikes which include the Straight Thrust Punch, the Vertical Back Knuckle, the Inverted Hammerfist, the Roundhouse Punch, and the Hammerfist Strike. Figure 95 concludes this illustration of the Master Key Set Striking Set One.

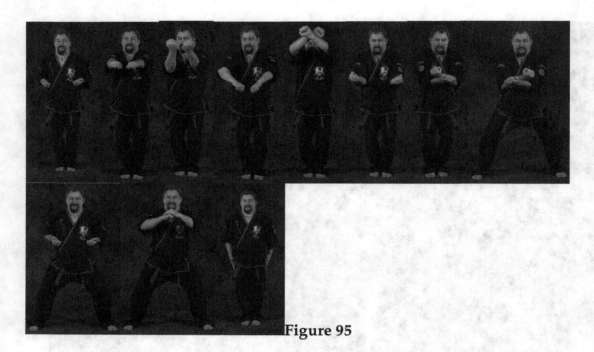

Figure 95

Master Key Sets explored in this volume include Blocking Set One and Striking Set One. These sets are elaborated upon and explained as they are taught within the Wu Shen Pai system. The sets are acknowledged as being **Master Key Sets** because they contain **Master Key Patterns**, **Master Key Basics**, **Master Key Concepts**, and other forms of **Master Keys**. In truth, they are the solution to a multitude of dilemmas. They give the Kenpo practitioner the keys to unlock a number of doors with their motion. They teach the practitioner about motion through the application of the movements and they serve to model concepts and principles that are foundational in the system.

Chapter Eight: Master Key Motion Patterns

Master Key Patterns

There are a number of patterns of motion which have been illustrated throughout this volume that are considered **Master Key Motion Patterns** within Wu Shen Pai Kenpo. These are, among others, the **Heart Shaped Pattern**, the **Half Heart Shaped Pattern**, the **Elliptical Circle**, the **Wave**, the **Tear Drop Pattern**, the **Figure Eight**, and the **Circle**, the **Square**, and the **Triangle**.

The **Heart Shaped Pattern** is first observed in the Wu Shen Pai Orange Belt technique **Grip of Death**. In the initial move of the technique, the opponent is struck simultaneously to the groin and the left kidney. This strike is executed in the **Heart Shaped Pattern**. The right hand describes the right side of the pattern, while the left hand describes the left side of the pattern. The result of employing this pattern in striking is to enhance the power of the strike by employing three-dimensional hitting. That is, hitting with height, depth, and width.

The **Half Heart Shaped Pattern** is seen in the extension to the technique Thrusting Salute, among other places. It is the single-handed version of the Heart Shaped Pattern. It is used for the same purpose, to obtain greater power and penetration in the strike. When the **Half Heart Shaped Pattern** is used in executing a strike, the effect realized is to obtain the use of all three dimensions in our motion. The model for this Master Key Pattern is the Wu Shen Pai Purple

Belt technique Parting Wings. In this technique, following the double blocks in the first move of the technique, the right hand executes a right Sword Hand strike to the floating rib. This strike is executed in a **Half Heart Pattern**.

The **Elliptical Circle** is used to extend the circle of a strike so as to impact multiple targets or leave multiple impressions on the opponent. One example of the Elliptical Circle is in the execution of the Inward Back Knuckle Rake in the Wu Shen Pai Yellow Belt technique Mace of Aggression. This sequence is illustrated in Figure 96 below.

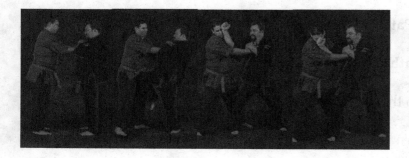

Figure 96

The **Wave** is observed for the first time when executing the elbow strike in the Yellow Belt Technique Mace of Aggression. The **Wave** represents a rounded edge best resembling a parenthesis. The **Wave** represents body mechanics, not the pattern of motion in the arm. It is so named since it resembles an ocean wave in the pattern of the movement and, like the ocean wave, possesses the potential for generating tremendous force. The body movement, when seen from above, would appear to be like a parenthesis. This motion, when executed properly, adds **Back Up Mass** to the motion of an elbow sandwich or elbow strike as it impacts the target. It is a method whereby the body mass is moved horizontally to effect its presence in a strike which is effected from the same dimension. It is seen in the pattern of movement for the body when the elbow sandwich to the opponent's head is executed. Figure 97 shows the execution of the Wave in this context.

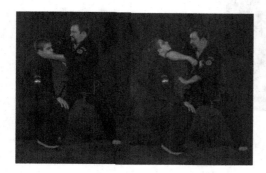

Figure 97

The **Tear Drop Pattern** is seen when we execute the technique Leaping Crane, among others. When we strike in this technique, we do so with penetration. This is the principle advantage of the Tear Drop Pattern. It allows us to strike a target with greater penetration, while still retaining the flow and continuity of motion. One example of this occurs when we make the initial hand strike in Leaping Crane. In this context, the **Tear Drop Shape** occurs on a vertical plane of action. In this technique the right hand strikes, pin pointing to the ribs, with this pattern. The penetration results in broken ribs while the flow and continuity of motion to follow through remains undisturbed. This particular strike is reprised for us in the Master Key Form Short Form Two. In this context the striking pattern is also executed on the vertical plane of action. One instance in which the Tear Drop Shape is modeled on the horizontal axis is illustrated in the Wu Shen Pai Kenpo 1st Degree Brown Belt technique Thrusting Salute. The

portion of the extension that models this striking pattern is shown in Figure 98.

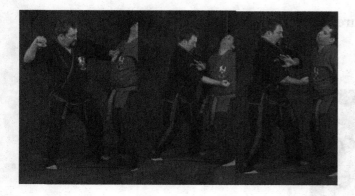

Figure 98

The **Figure Eight Pattern** acts as an additional check and a margin for

error when it is executed in our motion. It is seen in the Wu Shen Pai Orange

Belt technique Lone Kimono. This technique is illustrated in Figure 99 below.

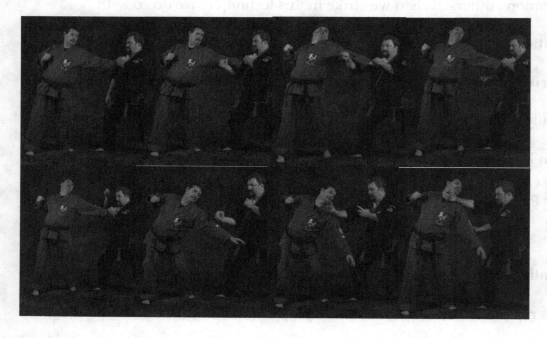

Figure 99

From the illustration in Figure 99, it is possible to observe the **Figure Eight master Key Pattern** in the context of this technique. In the event that the pin and the break are not executed in time to delay or stop the opponent from punching with the right hand, the clearing action and the follow up to the hand sword with your right hand act as an Inward Block to check the action of the punch. The Figure Eight is used in a different sense in the Wu Shen Pai Blue Belt technique Snaking Talon. Initially taught as a single hand **Figure Eight Pattern**, the technique's initial movements create broad coverage zones so as to capture and check the opponent's pushing hands. When taught at the advanced levels as a two hand **Figure Eight Pattern**, the same zone coverage is initiated, although the speed and explosion are increased measurably.

Also included in our understanding of Master Key Patterns is the **Circle**. The **Circle** may take many forms in our art. The simplest form is the Circle itself. This is expressed in a variety of Wu Shen Pai techniques. For example, there are **Interlocking Circles** which we observe in the Wu Shen Pai Kenpo techniques Flashing Wings, Flashing Mace, and Shield and Mace. The extensions for these techniques, taught in the Wu Shen Pai system at the 2nd Degree Black Belt level, also contain **Interlocking Circles** when we scrutinize the movement patterns of the lower body specifically the feet and legs. There are also **Kissing Circles**. These are Circles that do not interlock but touch each other at the perimeter. This form of the **Master Key Pattern** is also demonstrated in a number of techniques.

There is also the **Master Key Pattern** of the **Square**. This pattern is found in many techniques at the embryonic levels of learning footwork. Later this embryonic motion with the feet is rounded off for efficiency to form an **Elliptical Circle**. The **Square** as a **Master Key Pattern** typically allows us a **Margin for Error**. It is also a pattern that we learn and understand with greater ease at the **Primitive** or **Embryonic Phases** of motion when we are first learning to **Block Print**. Once we learn to use **Cursive Writing**, we discard our understanding of **Block Printing**, useful now only as a means of teaching others to write. So it is with the martial arts. We observe it for the first time in Blocking Set One in the transition from the Upward Block to the Inward Block. Dividing a **Square** into two equal parts creates a **Triangle**, yet another **Master Key Pattern**. Figure 100 shows the segment of **Blocking Set One** in which the **Square** is modeled.

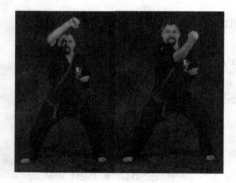

Figure 100

The **Triangle** as a **Master Key Pattern** might be found to contain useful applications for both the upper and lower body. As a point of reference, it serves to alert us to the body's vulnerable points. Key nerve centers and arteries of the body are located along the points of four triangles, located at the intersection of the arms and legs, while the pressure points impacting the nerves are found at a ninety degree angle to the limbs. The Triangle also serves to protect us. An **Open Ended Triangle** acts as a geometric protection against incoming attacking limbs. It serves to funnel incoming blows to a point where they can be intercepted and neutralized. The **Triangle** also serves, at an **Embryonic Stage of Motion**, as a reference point for stepping and footwork. This is later refined into more direct, circular steps.

These **Master Key Patterns of Motion** are modeled in our Self Defense Techniques, our Forms and Sets, and even in our Fundamental Basics in the Wu Shen Pai Kenpo system. They serve to alert us to motion patterns that enhance our efficiency, our flow and continuity, and our power in the execution of our techniques. Their study is but one more piece of the puzzle that enables us to further our self-mastery of our body in motion.

Chapter Nine: Mental Master Keys

Mental Master Keys

Within Wu Shen Pai Kenpo there is a point where the formal study of the art requires that we delve beyond the purely physical. There are **Master Key Concepts** that are so central to the study and practice of this art, that without these concepts playing an active role in the motion of the system, it may even be asserted that Wu Shen Pai Kenpo is not being practiced. Moreover, without an understanding of these deeper **Mental Master Keys**, it would be impossible to truly become a Black Belt in Wu Shen Pai. One example of a **Master Key Principle** is the principle of **Circular Compression**. This principle is one that was developed within Wu Shen Pai Kenpo thought and has been taught to the students of that art for over 10 years. To understand this principle and how it might assist you in maximizing your power, it is necessary only to insert this principle into a technique such as Five Swords. Compressing the circles within this technique would lead to greater speed, greater power, and generate exponential force from the additional assist gained from **Elastic Recoil**, yet another **Mental Master Key Principle**. Imagine performing the initial blocks and strikes within Five Swords in such a way that instead of a circle from the block to the point of impact, there would instead be an elliptical circle. This would cut the distance to the target as well as increase the speed and power gained from the ricocheting with the right hand and rebounding with the left hand. Another place where this principle would be applied would be in the technique Shielding Hammer. Initially, this technique is taught with somewhat large circles. As the student progresses in our system, they are taught increasingly concentric circles, or more accurately, the principle of **Circular Compression** is applied. As the circle of the elbow strike grows increasingly tight, devastating power is unleashed. Although these two techniques are often used to model the principle, Circular Compression may be employed in every technique in the system.

There are **Mental Master Keys** that would include **Economy of Motion, Meeting Force, the Presence and Use of Physical Master Keys, Anatomical Positioning, Point of Origin**, and **Timing for Effect.**

Economy of Motion involves utilizing the most efficient path or line to the target. It involves purposeful action with purposeful effect. It also involves **Efficiency of Action**. This principle, stated simply, is that method is best where maximum effect is achieved with minimum effort. Without **Economy of Motion** and its corollary principles including **Efficiency of Action**, Kenpo motion could not be said to be governed by modern concepts and theories. **Point of Origin** is another axiomatic principle that is directly linked to **Economy of Motion**. Like **Efficiency of Action, Point of Origin** is present in each movement of each technique. It simply states that the end of each individual action within the technique is the beginning point for the initiation of the next action. **Point of Origin** is related to **Economy of Motion** in that, should we violate principle of

Point of Origin, we would not be moving with **Economy of Motion** and would be violating that principle as well. **Economy of Motion** and its two corollary sub-principles **Efficiency of Action** and **Point of Origin**, taken together, are essential for one to claim to be practicing Wu Shen Pai Kenpo. They each must be present in each individual movement of each technique.

Meeting Force is yet another axiomatic, or ever present, principle of Wu Shen Pai Kenpo. **Meeting Force** is the method by which power is doubled when striking a target. Simply stated, **Meeting Force** is where the target is set in motion in the direction of the next strike. This, allowing for an angle of Incidence, means that the force of the strike meets the target moving toward the strike. The result is doubling the effective impact force of the strike. This principle, ideally, is present in all physical movements of the Wu Shen Pai Kenpo system.

The **Presence and Use of Physical Master Keys** is an essential pre-requisite to the practice of the Wu Shen Pai system of Kenpo. The **Physical Master Keys** have been the subject of discussion in all of the chapters in this work. The presence of these **Physical Master Keys** in the system are indisputable and their use is merely the application of one of our central axioms of training. It is important to train hard, train regularly, and train intelligently. If this is done, then no excuses will be necessary in the final analysis.

Anatomical Positioning, another axiomatic principle, has to do with the proper positioning of the opponent so that maximum efficiency is achieved when fitting the target of the next strike to the next weapon to be used. Put simply, Anatomical Positioning is where each successive strike or kick sets up the target to be impacted by the next strike or kick. The analogy to training, which might be drawn, has to do with the pool player who uses each of his successful shots to set up the next one.

Timing for Effect has to do with the **Rhythmic Timing** utilized in each technique for it to reach maximum effectiveness. There are Master Key Timing Patterns within the art, and within each technique, for maximum **Efficiency of Action**. There are **Five Master Key Timing Drills**. This will be the subject of a forthcoming video series on the art of Wu Shen Pai Kenpo. In addition to the **Master Key Timing Drills**, there are drills for each technique. For example, there are three timing drills associated with Delayed Sword. Two timing drills are associated with Alternating Maces, One with Deflecting Hammer, and Three with Sword of Destruction. As might be imagined, with 156 base techniques within the striking system of Wu Shen Pai Kenpo, there are hundreds of drills that have to do with timing and the performance of the self-defense techniques. In addition, **Timing for Effect** has to do with not merely blindly following one timing pattern, but rather utilizing the most efficient timing pattern for the technique sequence.

Master Key Theories include the **Power Equations** and **Family Groupings** that have already been discussed in Chapter One.

Master Key Strategies and Tactics

Master Key Strategies for dealing with an attack are also taught in Wu Shen Pai. There are, when confronting weapons in flight, **Five Master Key Strategies** for dealing with an attack. These strategies are rehearsed with respect to the initial movements in an attack and your own initial defense. These strategies are, in no particular order of importance, Inside, Outside, Underneath, On Top Of, and In Between. For example, the **Strategies** as they relate to a two hand front push are as follows. The model for Inside on a front two hand push is the Purple Belt technique Parting Wings. The Outside model is the Purple Belt technique Hooking Wings. The variable On Top Of is modeled by the Yellow Belt technique Alternating Maces. Underneath is assessed by the Blue Belt technique Thrusting Wedge, while In Between is modeled by the Blue Belt technique Snaking Talon. Against a front right hand step through punch The Inside model is the Orange Belt technique Five Swords. The Outside model is the Purple Belt technique Leaping Crane, while the On Top Of model is the Orange Belt technique Raining Claw. Underneath is modeled by the Green Belt technique Circles of Protection while In Between is modeled by the Green Belt technique Taming the Mace. These are merely examples of how we might assess the Five Master Key Strategies in the context of a weapon in flight. This would apply whenever a hand or arm is extended.

There are other Master key Strategies we analyze in Wu Shen Pai Kenpo. These have to do with being grabbed by two hands from the front or rear.

Whenever this occurs, the **Master Key Strategy** is to step off to the 45 Degree Angle in order to weaken one hand in the grip. The other hand then becomes a weaker single hand grab from which escape is more readily managed. This is called the **Pursuing the Diagonal Line**.

There are two **Master Key Tactics** as well. These are **Neutralizing the Angle of Opportunity** and **Checking Out the Zones of Offense**. This is simply related to body position. We seek to position ourselves, as soon as possible in the conflict, into a position relative to the opponent where we have closed the **Angle of Entry**. In other words, we want to have positioned ourselves in such a way that the opponent will have to work around their own hips and shoulders to strike us with the rear hand or leg, while the front hand and leg are checked out. A secondary **Master Key Tactic** is called **Checking Out.** This is to strike and block in such a way as to **Check Out** the **Height, Width, and Depth** of the opponent's **Zones of Offense**. We might observe not only how a Master Key technique models the various concepts and principles for our use, but we might also observe the **Master Key Strategies** and **Master Key Tactics** at work. Figures 101 through 103, examines the technique Attacking Mace in the Wu Shen Pai Yellow Belt curriculum. Included in the analysis is an assessment of some of **the Master Key Principles and Concepts** introduced through this technique. Also included in the analysis are some of the **Master Key Strategies and Tactics** which are used in this technique.

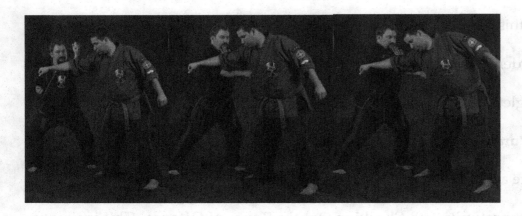

Figure 101

Stepping Back into a left Neutral Bow as the opponent throws a right step through punch, executing a right Inward Block cancels the width of the opponent so that he cannot effectively follow up with a left punch. The Master Key stance is taught here along with a Master Key Block. We have closed the angle of entry by stepping into a Left Neutral Bow as we stepped back. In addition, this technique teaches the Master Key Method of Execution Hammer and eventually teaches the Wu Shen Pai student to graft this to Thrust. We are operating along the Master Key Movement as we execute our block. In this case, it is the Master Key Movement, Left Side, Clockwise. Since we have earlier covered the opposite side in the curriculum with the initial moves of Delayed Sword, this technique serves to introduce Reverse Motion and review the concept of Opposite Motion. For every movement, concept, theory, or definition in Wu Shen Pai Kenpo there is an opposite and a reverse. This is what gives the art its balance. Turning into a Forward Bow, yet another Master Key Stance, we check the arm continuously to cancel the width zones and execute a right thrust punch to the ribs, striking the nerve centers between the 5th and 7th Intercostal Nerves. We emphasize the principle of the Bracing Angle as we throw the punch.

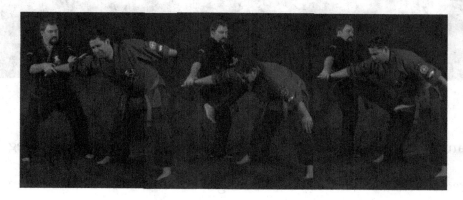

Figure 102

Utilizing the left hand to initiate a left hand heel palm strike, the elbow is broken and the strike results in continued cancellation of the width zones. The Angles of Entry are still cancelled. The Master Key Strategy and Tactics are being pursued. We have positioned ourselves in such a way continually throughout the technique so that the opponent will have to work around his own hips to kick with the rear leg or his shoulders to strike with the rear hands. The Snap Roundhouse Kick to the groin ensures that the opponent is Checked Out since cancellation of the Height Zones of Offense and Cancellation of the Width Zones of Offense mean that the opponent is completely Checked Out since the third Dimension, Depth, is automatically nullified.

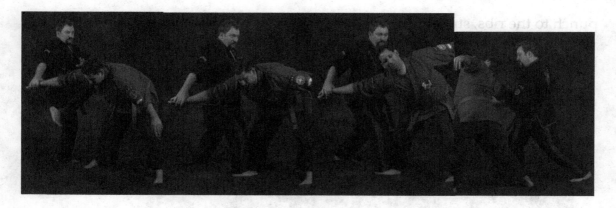

Figure 103

The replant of the kicking leg again closes the **Angle of Entry** and the leg is **close contoured** to maintain a check on the **height zones of offense**. The arm is locked at the elbow against the hip and this serves to maintain the check on the **width zones of offense**. An inverted punch thrusts into the lower portion of the ribcage thus employing a **bracing angle**. **Contouring** and **Complimentary Angles** are employed throughout. With the abundance of fundamental concepts and principles contained within this technique, it is easy to understand how it could be perceived as a Master Key technique.

Mental Master Keys are the means by which the practitioner of Wu Shen Pai Kenpo comes to understand the underlying principles inherent in Martial Arts training. It is Spiritual Master Keys, on the other hand, that help to establish the moral and ethical basis for the art which we practice.

Chapter Ten: Spiritual Master Keys

Spiritual Master Keys

There is a Chinese saying that one must first learn civility before he learns the art, and one must first know his ethics before he knows his skills. Civility here refers to good manners, courtesy, respect and consideration for others. Ethics, on the other hand, consists of a fundamental set of acceptable behaviors which codify the spirit of the martial arts and which the practitioner can rely on to guide their everyday actions and judgment in order to serve the ends of cultivating the body, mind, and spirit of the practitioner. Ethics is an indivisible part of the study of Wu Shen Pai Kenpo and the martial arts in general. Embracing an ethical code establishes certain moral guidelines for martial artists. Ethical principles serve as traditional, cultural, and social standards, or touchstones, through which practitioners are trained in Wu Shen Pai Kenpo. Central to these principles is the concept of nonviolence, respect for oneself and others, loyalty to one's family and country, and the following of the natural way. The adherence to a code of ethics affirms our moral obligation to our society and our fellow man. The concept of an ethical code embraces the attitudes, lifestyle, and the social and moral behavior of the practitioner. An ethical code enables us to evaluate the manner in which we behave in both word and action. A practitioner of Wu Shen Pai is not only a superior athlete, well-versed in combat, but also an upstanding citizen with good moral and social virtues. Fulfilling

ethical principles is both the true spirit and the ultimate goal of living the martial

way. It inspires all of us to continually strive for perfection within ourselves.

Ethics in Wu Shen Pai Training

Wu Shen Pai, in its literal translation from the Chinese means "martial

spirit family." Martial spirit is taken, in this context, to mean embracing a

lifestyle that we choose to term "living the martial way." Traditionally, the study

of Wu Shen Pai Kenpo consists of both the practice of skills and adherence to a

code of ethics and conduct. The skills learned from Wu Shen Pai Kenpo practice

hone our physical bodies; sharpen our reflexes and strengthen our resolve and

they should be counterbalanced by an equivalent honing of our spirit through

right action or conduct. The philosophy of Wu Shen Pai Kenpo enables us to

achieve harmony in society individually by living the fundamental tenets of

peace, wisdom, morals, love and self-discipline in our everyday lives. The

primary goal of learning Wu Shen Pai Kenpo is to become a better person who

lives within a greater set of expectations than does society at large. Living a

sincere life in balance becomes the prospect for those who adhere to the ethical

codes of the martial arts. Balance in life requires having a healthy balance in

both mental and physical terms. The art of Wu Shen Pai Kenpo cannot exist

without the spiritual aspect of our training. Without this aspect of our system,

our lives would be in perpetual imbalance, and our relationships would suffer from this instability. It is on this foundation that physical, emotional, and mental benefits derived from physical training are built. Our art is much more than just a workout. It is an alteration, both physically and mentally, of our lifestyle that will last a lifetime. We seek to bridge the gap between actions and thoughts, integrating our fighting skills with our philosophy.

Any worthwhile accomplishment requires a certain amount of dedication, effort, and discipline. This is no less evident in Wu Shen Pai Kenpo training. Every aspect of Wu Shen Pai Kenpo requires the harmonization of the mind, body, and spirit. This harmonization is achieved through mental focus and concentration combined with proper respiration and accurate physical techniques. The ultimate aim of Wu Shen Pai Kenpo training is the welfare of the practitioner. Self-defense skills should certainly be attained, but the focus should be on the development of the individual character of the practitioner. A well-rounded personality can only be realized if the spirit of the practitioner is right. Therefore the main goal in Wu Shen Pai Kenpo practice is to cultivate mind and body as one. We should not seek to use our training as a means to vent our anger, frustration or emotional problems. As serious Wu Shen Pai Kenpo practitioners, we should accept a philosophy of non-violence - a physical confrontation should be avoided whenever possible. The use of force is condoned only in self-defense or in the defense of the weak, the helpless, and the oppressed. Our philosophy does not condone meaningless rivalry, foolish stunts, intimidation of others, violent behavior, criminal activities, vanity, or any other vices or addictions. The Wu Shen Pai Kenpo practitioner displays this courage in the use of his skills to satisfy the demands of ethics, and in defense of his country or fellow human beings against unjust violence, to the point of supreme self-sacrifice, if necessary. The Wu Shen Pai Kenpo practitioner should use his knowledge only to protect himself and others from harm, and then only to the extent absolutely necessary to protect and remove himself from the situation. If it is necessary to use Wu Shen Pai Kenpo against an adversary, the practitioner should continue to use self-restraint and good judgment. A properly trained Wu Shen Pai Kenpo practitioner will do everything possible to avoid a physical confrontation, not only because he knows that such a confrontation is unnecessary, but also because he knows that he has a better than average chance of successfully defending himself and because a physical confrontation is philosophically degrading, as it indicates that all other means of avoidance have failed. Thus, the Wu Shen Pai Kenpo practitioner would adopt an attitude of self-control. He must bend like the willow. This discipline will help make him or her a better person and, at the same time, help him avoid unnecessary confrontations. It is the inner peace and confidence that the Wu Shen Pai practitioner develops that makes this possible. Patience is the key.

The History of Ethical Codes

There are those who reject the notion of a code of ethics and conduct as resting outside of the modern 20th Century notion of purely physical training and

166

skill development. Our personal lives, these critics would say, fall outside of the purview of our training. Still, such a view, and an emphasis, is not only unbalanced but also historically distorting for those who truly embrace a warrior lifestyle and train in the martial way. The modern lifestyle of the warrior in training embraces a code of conduct, a code of ethics, and principles for living and training that are not inherently different or divergent from those practicing an active warrior lifestyle in other cultures and arts in the past. Warriors have, throughout history, belonged to an elite group. Their conduct, as part of that group, has always been subject to observation and regulation since they have typically held a power of life over death that was unique within their societies. There were, for example, the Korean Hwarang. The Korean word that defines them is roughly translated as the "flower of manhood." This group of youthful warriors was credited with being the driving force that united the Korean peninsula under Silla rule. The Korean Hwarang embraced what might arguably be the earliest code of ethics and conduct. The Korean Hwarang, a group of young nobles trained in the cultural and the martial arts, were expected to adhere to a simple code of conduct known as the Hwarang O Kae or the Five Rules of the Hwarang. When the Hwarang flourished on the Korean peninsula, these five rules were accompanied by the Hwarang Kyo Hoon or the nine virtues of the Hwarang. The nine virtues are **Humanity, Justice, Courtesy, Wisdom, Trust, Goodness, Virtue, Loyalty, and Courage.** These five rules and nine virtues are today the root of Wu Shen Pai codes of conduct and discipline. It is also still utilized by many Korean martial arts as a code of ethics and conduct for their students and instructors. Other arts take a more specific approach to the formation of such codes. The feudal Samurai warriors of Japan also practiced a code of ethics and conduct which was based on self denial, restraint, and honor. The seven principles of the Code of Bushido or "the way of the warrior" were humility, truthfulness, bravery, benevolence, compassion, sincerity, loyalty and devotion to family, friends, and country. The Code of Bushido served as a constant reminder for the Samurai to perfect his character. His code of conduct, as we can observe, was not all that removed from that of the Hwarang. The code of the Samurai is still used today in modern Japanese business practices.

The Code of Ethics of Wu Shen Pai Kenpo

The Code of Ethics and the Code of Conduct inherent in the practice of Wu Shen Pai Kenpo is known, collectively, as Wu Wei. In the view of Wu Shen Pai Kenpo, codes of conduct and the underlying philosophies that form them are **Spiritual Master Keys** since they assist us in the formation of our attitudes and character. More accurately, it is perhaps our use of the **Spiritual Master Keys** that project into the **Code of Conduct** and the **Code of Ethics**. **Spiritual Master Keys** at the first level include **Being at Peace With Those Around You (Peace Without), Being at Peace With Yourself (Peace Within), and Having Confidence In Yourself.** All of these are rooted in the self-esteem of the practitioner. Building self-esteem and self-confidence is a hallmark of the training of every martial art. The primary purpose of training in Wu Shen Pai Kenpo is the cultivation of spirit and character. The training of real world self defense tactics is of grave importance, and this is not a responsibility that is taken lightly, but strict utility is not the primary purpose for training. It is still the main purpose and value of traditional martial arts to undertake the sculpting of human conduct and ethics or the formation of character.

This is addressed in Wu Shen Pai Kenpo through what is known collectively as the **Code of Ethics,** which has three components. The first of these is the **Code of Ethics** proper, dealing with the establishment of right purpose. This consists of the Nine Virtues and the Five Rules. There is also the **Code of Conduct,** aiding in the establishment of right conduct. Finally, there are **Nine Maxims of Training**. All of these, taken together, constitute the ethical core of Wu Shen Pai practice.

The notion of **Peace Within** is not accomplished outside of the practitioner's adherence to a **Code of Ethics**. A code of ethics is something which all warrior societies have agreed to adhere to. It is done often out of military necessity. However, it is also done for the benefit of the warrior, since it creates within the warrior a dividing line between conduct that is shameful and dishonorable and conduct that is acceptable. Peers will shun or ostracize those who violate these codes. Although such codes vary from culture to culture in minor ways, they share many similarities. The **Code of Ethics** in Wu Shen Pai is for the benefit of the practitioner in that it enables him or her to live at peace with himself. The Nine Rules are:

1) Humanity

Humanity is realized through compassion. Through intense training, the practitioner of Wu Shen Pai becomes quick and strong. He or she is not like other men or women. The Wu Shen Pai practitioner has developed, and is developing a power that must be utilized for the good of all. He or she has compassion, helping their fellow man at every opportunity. If an opportunity does not arise, then the Wu Shen Pai Practitioner goes out of his or her way to create an opportunity for service.

2) Justice

Seeking justice is a function of honesty. Be acutely honest in all your dealings with other people. Believe in justice, not from others, but arising from yourself. To the Wu Shen Pai practitioner there should be no shades of gray in the question of honesty and justice. There is only right and wrong. The battle between good and evil is not won by inaction. 'The only thing necessary for the triumph [of evil] is for good men to do nothing.' – Edmund Burke

3) Courtesy – Polite Courtesy

Respect and sensitivity toward others has a strong effect on all of our personal relationships, both at work or at school, and with friends and family. Along with respect for others, comes an awareness of others and their needs. Respect for those who are senior and from whom we learn is essential for learning. Without this basic element, the teacher can not teach and the learner can not learn. Practitioners of Wu Shen Pai should not only show etiquette for the seniority system and honor senior members but reflect self respect, respect for other practitioners, and respect for all human beings. A Wu Shen Pai Practitioner has no reason to be cruel. They have no need to prove their strength. They have nothing to prove to anyone. A practitioner of Wu Shen Pai is courteous, even to his enemies. Without this outward show of respect, we are nothing more than animals.

4) Wisdom

All who have great accomplishments in their life, also display great wisdom. The course of true wisdom is humility. This is because, without humility, no one is capable of learning. The more humble a person is, the more willing he is to learn. This is the prerequisite to the attainment of knowledge. Just as an empty cup can be readily filled, an open mind is sure to learn. There is an old Korean saying: Large egos are carried by small minds. A Wu Shen Pai practitioner seeks after knowledge, and its application, wisdom. The ultimate aim of Kenpo is where the Tiger is seen but the Dragon prevails.

5) Trust

Trust is given and trust is earned through a life of complete sincerity. A true martial artist must have a high moral character, be open, forthright and honest. He should never be intimidated by power, corrupted by money, nor weakened by unwholesome desires. A person must never be vain, but he can never be without pride. The true martial artist must have enough pride not to be used and corrupted by others, or lower oneself to grovel at the feet of the rich and powerful. The Wu Shen Pai practitioner will never permit himself to be used by an evil individual. The independence and integrity of personal character must be defended at all cost so that Wu Shen Pai as an art and its practitioners as individuals may stand tall under any circumstance. In doing so, one will always have a clear conscience and righteous strength. This is the physical manifestation of the martial spirit through merging the principles of the way and the art. When a practitioner of Wu Shen Pai has said that an action will be performed, it is as good as done. Nothing will stop him from completing what he has said he will do. The practitioner of Wu Shen Pai does not have to give his word or promise. Complete Sincerity is a function that leads to trust.

6) Goodness

Doing what is right in the sight of men and God. Seeking after that which is pure, moral, and ethical; that which is good. More than mere actions, goodness involves purity of motive as well as right action. Thus right intention is fused with action to balance the scales of morality and ethics

7) Virtue

Virtue is realized through adherence to honor. This is, in turn a function of duty fulfilled. A true Wu Shen Pai practitioner has only one judge of honor, and that is himself. Decisions that are made and how these decisions are carried out are a reflection of yourself and a reflection of who you really are. You cannot hide from yourself. Your own wisdom should become sharply refined as you evaluate how your decisions are made.

8) Loyalty

When a practitioner of Wu Shen Pai has done something or said something, he or she owns responsibility for that thing. He or she is responsible for it and all the consequences that follow out of it. A Wu Shen Pai practitioner is immensely loyal to, and fiercely responsible for, those in his or her care. Loyalty is linked to duty and obligation.

9) Courage

The kind of courage that we speak of as a Wu Shen Pai practitioner is heroic courage. This is the willingness to stand up for truth and justice no matter the cost. This is a traditional virtue in Wu Shen Pai and the martial arts in general. The courage spoken of here is a higher kind of courage. It is the courage of self-sacrifice, of standing up for the truth, regardless of what the odds are or what the cost may be. It is not the petty bravery of proving one's self-worth by engaging in meaningless rivalry, foolish stunts or the intimidation of others. The courage in this sense is an important test of a person's true worth. In times of danger or crisis, a Wu Shen Pai practitioner must stand up and be counted. The willingness to sacrifice is the hallmark of a true martial artist. No human endeavor can ever be possible without some sacrifice. Heroic courage call on one to rise up above the masses of people who are afraid to act. Hiding like a turtle in a shell is not living at all. A Wu Shen Pai practitioner must have this kind of heroic courage. It is absolutely risky. It is dangerous. It is living life to its fullest. Life in this state is truly complete, full, and wonderful. Heroic courage is not blind courage; it is intelligent, active, and strong.

Taken together, the Nine Moral Precepts and the Five Rules of Wu Shen Pai form the Wu Shen Pai Kenpo Code of Ethics. These are: **Humanity, Justice, Courtesy, Wisdom, Trust, Goodness, Virtue, Loyalty, and Courage.** The Five Rules of Wu Shen Pai are:

1) **Loyalty to one's country.**

2) **Loyalty to one's parents and teachers.**

3) **Trust and Brotherhood among friends.**

4) **Courage – Never retreat in the face of the enemy.**

5) **Justice – never take life without cause.**

The **Code of Conduct**, an outgrowth of the **Code of Ethics**, also serves to create **Peace Within**. More importantly, however, the Code of Conduct establishes a basis for right action, and thus the basis of **Peace Without**. The **Nine Virtues** of the **Code of Ethics** should be a code for living which every Wu Shen Pai practitioner strives to uphold. Each student must affirm, accept and sign as binding, the following code of ethics. The following is our Wu Shen Pai **Code of Conduct**:

I hold sacred the inalienable right to all men and women to own and bare arms for the purpose of self-defense. I further hold that those who are trained in the ancient arts of self-defense take upon themselves obligations and responsibilities, which I now freely take upon myself. I therefore pledge the following:

- o That I shall never misuse my skill to hurt or make afraid.

- o That I shall fight if forced to defend myself, I shall be slow to anger, loathe to take offense, quick to forgive, and ever to forget personal affront.

- o That pride shall never rule my passions.

- o That I will defend with all the skill I possess the weak, the helpless, and the oppressed.

- o I pledge an unswerving loyalty to my instructor and those who have gone before.

o I pledge a continued effort to sharpen my skill, to increase my knowledge and to broaden my horizons.

o I understand that this rank I accept is that of a student and therefore I will be obligated to teach from time to time under the direction of my instructor in order to learn the skills of a teacher.

o I understand that I am but a beginner in a new, more responsible direction, that to retain this honor I must serve my fellow students and my fellow man.

o I understand that the private affairs of other students and instructors that come to my attention during the exercising of my responsibilities are privileged communications and must never be discussed with any living soul.

o I vow that I will never violate this code for the sake of personal profit

o I recognize the right and necessity for order and regulation within the Arts and accept the right of this Association to govern its own affairs by mutual consent.

o When speaking to those within this fraternity, I shall make no statement that will detract in any way from the fame or reputation of any of my fellows.

o When speaking of those belonging to another system or a different Art, I shall strive to say only those things I know to be fact, avoiding with all diligence any hearsay and gossip.[1]

This Code of Conduct forms the basis for finding Peace Without. Both the **Code of Conduct** and the **Code of Ethics** are an outgrowth of **Peace with God**. If one is unable to make **Peace with God**, then theoretically, it is difficult to imagine one who is able to either find **Peace Within** or to be at **Peace Without**. Both aspects of our Spiritual growth find their root within our relationship with our creator.

Peace with God stems from obedience to His code of Ethics and Conduct. It is in loving others and in loving Him (God) that we define our own self-esteem. Finally, Self Confidence is rooted in self-knowledge with its emphasis on certain Training Maxims, that, if followed, will invariably lead to increased capability.

Training Hard, Training Regularly, and Training Intelligently are but the outward manifestations of these inner **Training Maxims**. These are:

- ➢ Correctness in Attitude

- ➢ Excellence in Training

- ➢ Directness in Action

- ➢ Effectiveness in Combat

---

[1] With thanks to the Whipping Willow Association and the National Chinese Kenpo Karate Association from whom this Code of Conduct was adapted. Also notable are the excerpts from the various creeds of the International Kenpo Karate Association.

- Humility in Heart

- Strength in Character

- Freedom in Expression

- Thirst for Knowledge

- Power in Truth

- Respect in Wisdom

The Wu Shen Pai **Code of Ethics** and its accompanying **Code of Conduct** embody the same elements that have been present in all such similar codes embraced by warrior societies and cultures around the world. Loyalty, Honor, Integrity, Discipline, Trust, Courage, Justice, Compassion, Wisdom, and Goodness are embraced not because they are a means to an end, although they are, but because these traits are an end unto themselves. These traits are what we, as warriors, seek because it is in the pursuit of these traits that the practitioner's character is molded. It is in the pursuit of these traits that we ultimately seek the unattainable, human perfection. Training becomes, in this worldview, a means to the end of cultivation of the human character and the attainment of the highest levels of human physical, mental, and emotional achievement. It is the pursuit of excellence in which we are engaged. This is ultimately the purpose of codes of conduct, and of ethical and procedural norms within a training society. We also willingly submit ourselves to our martial arts societies and organizations through these codes of conduct and ethical standards in an effort to maintain accountability to our art, our master instructors, and our community. American Kenpo of the 60's and 70's is growing and developing into the art that will meet the needs of the 21st Century. Wu Shen Pai Kenpo was developed and will be there in the future of Kenpo to fill the needs of today and tomorrow. The strength of our art and its leadership in morals, ethics, and the sense of family and heritage will be the keys to the growth of our new American Wu Shen Pai Kenpo Karate system.

Afterward

The theories advanced in this book are wholly a part of the Wu Shen Pai Kenpo Karate system. This is not to say that some systems of martial arts or that some systems of Kenpo other than my own, do not embrace these ideas and theories. I cannot represent these arts, only my own. Therefore, no attempt is made to do so. This book is part of a three-volume set. Volume Two will cover the joint manipulation aspects, or the chin na, of Wu Shen Pai Kenpo. Volume Three of Advanced Kenpo Karate, the Wu Shen Pai Method will examine the Pressure Point and Cavity Press Theories as they are applied in this system. The art of Wu Shen Pai Kenpo is regulated through the International Kenpo Karate Society. This association has as its emblem a crest which is visible within this and future volumes. Below is an illustration of that crest and some of its meaning.

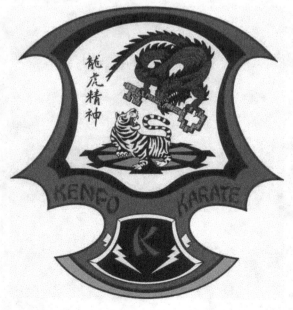

The Shape: The topmost portion of the crest is shaped like a roof that gives shelter to all who come under it. The SIDES {)(} are curved conversely because like the roof of a Chinese home they are to send evil back to where it came from, whenever it tries to descend. The representation of a Tora gate in the crest, which is the interior black shape, represents the entry into the gateway of knowledge. Within this gateway, the Tiger and the Dragon exist. The sides also represent the separate halves of the heart shape. The bottom part of the crest above the axe represents the teardrop pattern, while the shape resting above that one represents the "wave" pattern of energetic pulsing. This is a pattern of motion that enables us to obtain a greater understanding of the body mechanics behind various movements as we execute certain short range strikes. The bottom forms the shape of an ax - it represents the executioner. In the event a member is influenced by evil ideas and thoughts contrary to our philosophy, or shames the I.K.K.S. as an organization, he is cut off, never to co-exist with us again. The outline of the axe is represented in two ways. First, what is represented by the bottom of the crest. Second, that which is represented by interior of the bottom of the crest. This represents forward and reverse motion and black dot focus. The interior of the bottom of the crest appears to be three dimensional. This is symbolic of three-dimensional hitting, or striking with the utilization of height, width, and depth. The four points in the crest represent the four ranges of combat. These are out of contact, in contact, contact penetration, and contact manipulation. The three top most points in the crest represent the three phases of motion, primitive, mechanical, and spontaneous. The three states of motion may also be represented in these three points. These three states of motion are the solid, liquid, or gaseous state. The three points of view might also be understood as being referenced by these three points on the crest. The shape of the crest above the axe represents the tear drop shape used in many Wu Shen Pai Kenpo techniques. Another line or shape utilized in our motion and represented in the crest shape is that of the half heart. These patterns, the wave, the teardrop shape, and the heart shape, are master key patterns that are utilized in the physical motions of our techniques.

The Tiger: Represents the earthly strength derived through the early stages of learning. This is the stage where the individual is more impressed with his or her own physical prowess. The tiger is looking upward toward the dragon, symbolic of the tiger seeking the wisdom and knowledge of the dragon. Within the tiger's tail is a Master Key Pattern, the elliptical circle.

The Circle: Is symbolic of several things. It depicts life itself, as a continuous cycle, where there is no beginning or end. So it is with the art of Kenpo. It too is a cycle of unending and perpetual movement or motion. Techniques follow a cycle, movements are part of a cycle. Physical prowess, humility, and self restraint are no more than components of a progressive learning cycle. The circle is the base from which our alphabet stems. It also depicts the continuous circle of friendship which should exist between the members of our association. (1) All moves evolve from a circle whether they are defensive or offensive. (2) The circle represents the bond of friendship that should continuously exist among Studio and Association members. The directional pattern upon which the Tiger and

Dragon rest are symbolic of all forms of motion and of our analysis of motion as Kenpo practitioners. The lines within the circle represent the linear aspects of the art fused with the circular. The lines within the pattern also represent the eight basic directions of attack and defense. The circle is the base from which our alphabet stems. The circle, with its dividing lines, forms the alphabets listed. The eight directions of attack and defense which form the roots of the universal Pattern is the base upon which the tiger stands.

The Oriental Writing: Is a reminder of the originators of our art, the Chinese. It is in respect to them and not that we serve them. The lettering to the Left means "Tiger Dragon Spirit Way" or the Spirit of the Tiger and the Dragon. It is symbolic of the spirit of martial training and of spiritual attainment which characterize our discipline and is a constant reminder that we want to attain the spiritual level and that the physical level is only a stepping stone, or vehicle, that we use to reach the higher or spiritual level. The spirit of the Dragon and the Tiger is indicative of our following the martial way, the path of the warrior. The letters exist between the tiger and leading to the dragon symbolic of our higher spiritual attainment as we reach that goal.

The "K" : stands for Kenpo, the art which we practice, or Karate. It may also signify Kindness.

The Colors: The white background signifies the many beginners who form the basis of the art. The yellow or orange represents the first level of proficiency, the mechanical stage, the dangerous stage of learning. It is a time when the student is more impressed with the physical, and who, like a freshman in college, thinks he knows all the answers. The angles of attack and defense are colored GRAY because it is symbolic of the brain -- the brain of our organization and the intelligence which exists in our system, since the brain has always been referred to as GRAY matter. This refers to the elements of logic and thought which are always central to the Wu Shen Pai Kenpo system. The gray at the bottom of the axe blade is symbolic of our continual sharpening of our natural weapons to a finely honed edge. This also represents the hope that we will always be in the forefront or at the cutting edge of the Kenpo system. This concept, as well as its opposite and reverse are found within the axe shape as well. The red exterior of the crest indicates the colors of professorship. They contain and control all that is within and act as protection against all that is without. This element is also present in the red color of the "K" and the red coloring to the dragon in the studio crest, symbolic of spiritual attainment. The red, black, and white in the layers of the central portion of the crest represent proficiency, achievement, and authority. Brown, the color of the tiger's eyes, represents the advanced students who are not great in number. The brown in the eyes also represents that, at this level, the student becomes more observant. His eyes, like that of the tiger, are keen, ever so watchful and critical, always looking up to the higher levels of proficiency, striving for perfection, preparing for the day when he or she will bear the label of expert. This level of expert proficiency is represented by the color Black. Red is the color associated with professorship over and above the black but yet, as indicated by the colors of the dragon, there are still traces of White in the dragon's eyeball, Yellow or Orange on the dragon's fins, Brown in the iris of the eyeball, and Black in the pupils of the eyeball. This is to remind even the professor that he too should always be so humble and be able to go back to any level, whatever it might be, and perform the things that he expects of others at these levels so as to never demand too much of his students. The black of the interior of the axe blade represents Black Dot Focus, or the total awareness of all around us, which our system teaches. The Black interior of the Upper Crest indicates the level at which we round off corners and elongate the circles of motion. The interior of the axe blade represents the elements of forward and reverse motion also. Opposites and dualities of motion and opposing forces are represented by the White and Black background of the crest.

THE DRAGON: represents spiritual strength which comes with seasoning. This mental attitude is attained during the individual's later years of training. It is placed above earthly strength (as indicated and observed on the patch) since the individual at this stage has learned to develop humility and self-restraint. He is holding the golden "master key" which is the basis of all wisdom and knowledge in Wu Shen Pai Kenpo.

THE DIVIDING LINES: In the circle represent: (1) the original eighteen hand movements - directions in which the hands can travel; (2) they are the angles from which you or an opponent can attack or defend; (3) form the pattern in which the feet too can travel - an explanation of the Universal Pattern will clarify this.

THE LIGHTNING BOLTS: Represent the explosive speed and power which our students are renowned for possessing. It represents our philosophy of obtaining and generating power and our philosophy of action when fighting. The angle at which they are held represents the triangle as a geometric pattern and the diagonal angle of scaption, central for the proper execution of our motion. Another Master Key pattern represented here is the open ended triangle, often used to trap or redirect motion.

MASTER KEY: Symbolizes that those who wear the crest of the International Kenpo Karate Society possess the true Master Keys to motion taught through the American Wu Shen Pai Kenpo System that enable us to ultimately decode and master all forms of motion. The Master Key is portrayed as a puzzle which is comprised of many pieces. This represents our view that the Master Keys to motion are many and take many forms within many differing contexts. Hidden within the Master Key is the cross which is symbolic of the Christian beliefs of our Association's founder, Peace with God being the Spiritual Master Key. The plus pattern is also part of the key, a geometric Master Key to understanding the art.

TAILS OF THE TIGER / DRAGON: Represents the elements of circularity of motion which our system contains. A figure 8 is hidden within the Dragon's tail symbolic of one of the many Master Key Patterns found within American Wu Shen Pai Kenpo. Interlocking Circles are also represented within both the tails of the Tiger and Dragon. The end of the Dragon's tail and the Tiger's tail represent the elements of forward and reverse motion. They also represent the opposite motion found within the system. We might also consider the Dragon's Tail to represent kissing circles, yet another master key pattern of motion. The Tiger's tail represents the elliptical circle, another Master Key Pattern.

This is but some of the meaning inherent in our Association Crest. It is my hope that this book has been enlightening, informative, and useful in your training, no matter which style or system that you might train in. It is my wish for you that your journey in the martial way be a long and a fruitful journey.

Printed in the United States
by Baker & Taylor Publisher Services